CW00485144

Tantric
Secrets

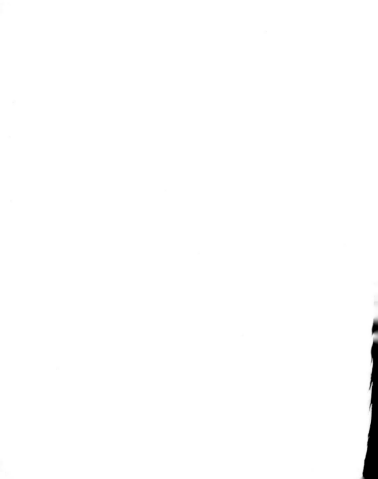

Tantric Secrets

7 Steps to the Best Sex of Your Life

Cassandra Lorius

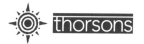

To Liz Dean, my marvellous editor

Thorsons
An Imprint of HarperCollins*Publishers*
77–85 Fulham Palace Road,
Hammersmith, London W6 8JB

The website address is: www.thorsons.com

and *Thorsons* are trademarks of
HarperCollins*Publishers* Ltd

First published by Thorsons 2003

5 7 9 10 8 6

Illustrator: Colin Hadley

A catalogue record of this book
is available from the British Library

ISBN 13 978–0–00–716606–0
ISBN 10 0–00–716606–0

Printed and bound in Thailand by Imago

Contents

Introduction

What is Tantra?

Tantra is an ancient path of self-development that regards sexual energy as the primary manifestation of our life force. This life force is a powerful current of energy that flows through us all. When you are in harmony, this energy is 'woven' with the energy of other people and all the life forms around us. The term 'Tantra' implies that we can weave all the different threads of our existence into a more satisfying whole. Through Tantra, you can experience love and sex as a flowing together of energies. Techniques that were once secret – only available to the initiated – are revealed here to rekindle your lust for life and regain a vibrant sense of self. By being more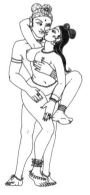

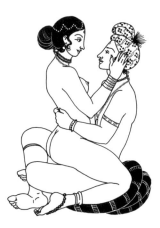

loving and connected in the ways in which you relate to your partner, you can create more fulfilling sex and a deep, loving intimacy. Tantra guides you through the gateway of lovemaking to open to spiritual bliss.

The message is simple: celebrate your relationship with a spirit of wonder and playfulness. Tantra is easy to grasp once you experience it – simply stop thinking and start feeling. Focus on the present moment, as you'll feel more vital when you wholeheartedly live in the 'now'. Be sensually aware of your body, and express your sense of aliveness and passion through it. Reconnecting with your body in a positive way via your senses gives you a surge of wellbeing and energy. Sexual energy is a fundamental indicator of your level of vitality. When you're feeling great, your body is vital and eroticized.

Tantra for your relationship: the seven steps to bliss

Tantra is a potent means of revitalizing your relationship. Cultivating Tantra means embracing a dynamic approach to sex, love and life in general that will fill you with bliss. The starting point of this process is to reaffirm the place of spirit in your life, and make space for a soul connection in your sexual relationship. A loving relationship encourages you to expand sexuality into a more integrated way of being. Tantric techniques teach you how to unlock your energy and use it to bring bliss into your lives.

The ethos of this book is opening your heart, filling your being with loving emanations and sweetening your relationship with love and compassion. *Tantric Secrets* reveals the seven chapters, or steps, that you can take to transform your relationship into one of bliss. Each Step explores issues appropriate to the unfolding of an integrated sexuality according to Tantric sources – including meditative exercises that you can use on your own path to fulfilment through sacred sex.

Tantric Secrets offers ideas for short practices to radically improve your experience of sex and open your heart to love and bliss. Cumulatively, they lead to a sensual bonk-fest, taking you into the realm of bliss. You can pick and choose according to what inspires you. However, I suggest that you do start by looking at Step 1, because the secret of maintaining a loving relationship is to love yourself. In these demanding times, many of us lead stressful lifestyles that hamper our free spirits, making it difficult to delight in our sensual natures.

To prepare to deepen your relationship, begin by de-stressing both mind and body. In **Step 1** you nurture both body and soul. You learn to love yourself by taking care of your needs; when you nurture yourself, you have the resources to nurture others. Learn to treat your own body with respect, remembering that your body is a temple dedicated to life and love.

When you have activated the energy of body and soul in your own being, you are free to reach out toward your partner with an open heart.

In **Step 2,** you connect with your lover as an energy-body, relating to each other at the level of your inner core rather than your surface personalities.

In **Step 3,** you stimulate your sensuality through rituals that enliven all your senses. Ritual is about inviting the sacred into your life. It is this sense of sacredness that helps you to step beyond your normal limits, into a closer connection with your partner. If you associate activities like lighting candles and incense with an attitude of receptivity to the sacred dimension, each time you do this you enter into a Tantric frame of mind.

To awaken your sexual energy and access your passionate nature, **Step 4** explores your desire, and includes physiological exercises that combine strengthening your love muscle with breathing and visualization exercises.

Step 5 involves sexual healing, and clearing difficult emotions that may be blocking the flow of energy in your relationship. Communication needs to underpin your sexual relationship in order for it to be close and loving.

You work on your technical abilities as a lover in **Step 6,** learning to pleasure yourself and your lover, exploring your orgasmic potential and lengthening and deepening your orgasms so that you can both have multiple orgasms. For women, discover how clitoral and g-spot stimulation is crucial to sexual satisfaction. For men, learning to defer gratification develops the potential for much greater orgasmic pleasure.

Step 7 makes sex sacred by incorporating the powerful Tantric techniques of breathing and visualization to move energy through your being during lovemaking. Together, you create a joint body of energy united in sexual bliss – an experience that opens you to the Tantric awareness that bliss is the nature of life itself.

What is Tantric meditation?

In Eastern traditions, meditation is seen as the royal road to nurturing the soul. The secret wisdom of Tantra shows you how to forge a meditative approach to sex, which gives it transcendent power. Soulful sex becomes a pathway to direct experience of the divine realm of love, which Tantra describes as joyful bliss. In weaving the lover's path with your partner, you make connections between heart, spirit and body to bring the spiritual dimension firmly into your life.

You unite your two beings in divine love and align this love with the natural flow of love in the universe during lovemaking.

Tantric meditation induces a state of deep, dynamic relaxation in which you remain very engaged with the world around you. Relaxation involves letting go of struggle in life and surrendering to the flow of energy through your being. In dynamic relaxation, you recover a life-affirming attitude – joy, spontaneity and the sensual pleasure of life.

This dynamic state is also passionate; it's full of lust for life and love for others, a deep expression of your core eroticism rather than a superficial sexual orientation. It is not about tarting up your relationship with exotic stimulation, but about going more deeply into the loving connection that already exists. As you tune into your partner, so your relationship deepens. You affirm your lover's inner beauty by loving them as much as yourself.

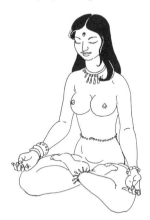

Through Tantric meditation, you also rediscover the innocence and playfulness in your partnership.

Develop awareness

Meditation is the heart of the Tantric journey. Through meditation you become sensitive to the movements of energy in your own body and learn to see others as energy-beings. Ultimately, the awareness that grows through meditation, visualization and energy practices enables you to feel the vast energy flow that physicists describe as our fundamental reality. Through surrendering the belief that you are separate from other living beings, you can join in the dance of creation.

Take time every day to meditate. Meditation can be described as letting 'doing' fall away. One of the key practices that this book constantly emphasizes is simply paying full attention to whatever is occurring in the present moment. (That is why *Tantric Secrets* doesn't encourage sexual fantasies that take your concentration away from your partner and from what is happening between you.) Paying careful attention makes you more sensitive in your interactions and deepens the connections between you and your deeper self, as well as with others. Being more alive to your own experience helps you to fully immerse yourself in it, rather than stand outside your own life as a detached observer.

Become a witness

Meditation also encourages you to become more of a witness to your own life, so that you can perceive more clearly what is happening to you at the same time as being absorbed in it. As a witness to your own life you develop insight into how you relate, rather than hold yourself back from others because of a critical or judgmental attitude. In order to let go of such attitudes you need to open up to the transpersonal nature of love, which is unconditional. Let love flow through you.

Get closer to your partner

To create a nurturing and loving environment twenty-four hours a day, seven days a week, try to make time to touch base with your inner self each day through meditation or yoga *(see pages 25, 35)*. These practices help you to connect with your partner and activate your loving energy.

Many of us feel the need for greater closeness, yet with our busy lives we can find it almost impossible to dedicate time to relate with the degree of attention that real communication requires. Yet you can make time – it is the degree of connection with each other that is important, rather than the length of time spent together.

You can also make time by letting go of a sense of hurry; be fully present and emotionally available in the here and now. Reluctance to make time for closeness can arise from a feeling of resistance or fear about intimacy. This book offers techniques for breaking down defences against closeness and going to the heart of intimacy, both sexually and emotionally *(see Step 5, page 175)*.

Think of a period in your life when the world sparkled with promise, suffused with sensuality. Do you recall the delicious rush of anticipation you felt on seeing your lover walk towards you, feeling the warm thrill of their touch on your arm, or the elation of gazing directly into their eyes? If your erotic aliveness is more or less shut down, such sensations may only come in unexpected moments, when you're startled by undercurrents in a friendship or with a stranger. The tingling promise of eroticism is a reminder of our true nature, filling us with a surge of energy and delight – the original meaning of the word lust. You can allow this erotic electricity to remain subdued, or you can consciously choose to ignite it, both alone and with your partner.

A Tantric model for loving

Tantra has a sophisticated concept of love. In Western culture, love is often clichéd as romantic attraction built on fantasies and projections. In Tantra, you use love to connect with the essence of your partner.

A Tantric model has a lot to teach us about relationships. It sees relationships as a flow of energy and emotions as a form of energy. This approach offers you a radically different way of dealing with difficult emotions in your relationship. Tantra says that you are not your emotions or your mind – this is your false self. You are really an energy-field composed of dancing atoms. This understanding encourages you to drop your false self, no longer identifying yourself as the sum total of all your problems and emotions. As these negativities fall away, your true nature is revealed and you regain your natural state of presence, or 'being'. You can fully engage in the moment, rather than be withdrawn or preoccupied with old hurts, disappointments or insecurities that sap your energy. Just as children drop the past as soon as it is over and deal with what is right in front of them, you too can relearn the ability to constantly let go.

By letting go of inappropriate emotions and impossible expectations, we accept that we cannot determine our relationships with other people. Relationships are mysterious and ultimately unknowable. If you surrender to the greater power of the universe that is glimpsed in the heart of this mystery, you open your hearts to each other.

Tantra is all about dissolving your ego, learning to be receptive, opening your heart – letting love dissolve any

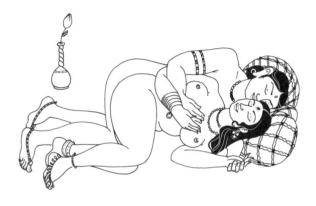

emotional negativity – and seeing the divine in every aspect of your life, including the divinity in your partner. It's about seeing the nature of the world as love, and making your relationship central to your life.

Body knowledge

A great way to side-step all the emotional problems that a relationship often activates is to encourage the wisdom of your body, allowing yourself to feel love and express it physically.

Traditional spiritual paths advocate cutting off from the body and disowning bodily experience, but Tantra regards your body as the gateway to your deepest self. A Tantric perspective invites you to abandon yourself to life, to enjoy your body and take pleasure in daily life. This means acknowledging the beauty of your sensory experience – attuning to nature, your own deeper nature and to those around you.

Some people are naturally Tantric. They are alive to the abundance of energy and sensitive to its subtle manifestations in their lives. They feel engaged and inspired in their relationship with the world around them – connected, perceptive, aware and sensitive. It is possible for us all to live like this, by uncovering our innate sensuality and opening to joy.

Tantra for healing

Love is the source of healing power, which emanates from the energy-body. An energy-body is the invisible energy within all of us *(see page 48)*. Once you accept the importance of love, you can use Tantra meditations to heal your energy-body and your emotional pain, and any sexual wounding and withholding that stems from a closed heart. Throughout this book there are meditations for healing, as well as meditations to expand your awareness of the subtle dimensions of life. These techniques create more harmony and happiness in your relationship, and enable you to explore your full sexual potential.

Seeing you, your partner and your relationship as bodies of energy helps you to open up to everyday experience, engaging with your own life in a transformative way. Changing your attitude in accordance with Tantra creates a radical shift of perspective – you see the joy in mundane activities. By making the imaginative leaps suggested in this book, you can remodel your world in the image of your dreams.

Tantra and sexuality

Sexuality is a powerful force that motivates us in many ways. Your libido is the source of your sexual energy, or *kundalini,* that can be awakened through arousing your sexual fire. You unblock and channel the potent energy attached to sexuality so that it is available to enliven your whole being. Your body can dance with sensual excitement.

Tantra uses the fire of your sexual passion to fuel spiritual growth. Sexuality is a dynamic expression of your psyche – more a state of consciousness than a biological drive. It enriches your relationships and your life.

The quality of attention and togetherness achieved during sex allows you to engage with your partner at a deep level of intimacy. Focus on opening your heart so that you can feel the love within your heart pouring out, and enjoy a deep sense of connection – both with your lover, and through them with the rest of the world.

Love yourself

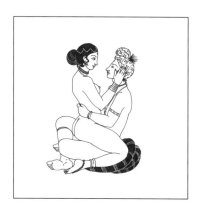

Take the first step to Tantric bliss by learning to love yourself. Before you can love your partner unstintingly, you must love yourself. Self-love is the key to self-development. Tantra deepens intimacy with your partner, but this means first taking responsibility for the quality of love that you can give. Look inside yourself to discover the depths of love. In Tantric sex, love is seen as a universal energy that is also inside you both individually. Through intimate lovemaking, you can explore and exchange this vital source of love.

If you lack confidence or are frequently emotionally demanding in a relationship, you risk becoming overly dependent on your partner; if you feel distant, you are likely to push your lover away. In order to be truly happy in a relationship, it is necessary to be joyful when you are alone.

You may, however, find it difficult at first to take the time you need to look after yourself. You may need to reframe your thinking, affirming that you are a worthwhile human being and that finding the path to love and bliss is a basic human right. Tantra says that love and self-love is your birthright. It is not selfish to nourish yourself, pursuing activities that feed you. If you are used to pleasing others at your own expense, take the space to do what you enjoy. First of all you may require time alone, getting to know yourself and what motivates you; you can do this by recognizing the positive activities that nourish you – gardening, walking, dance, music or other creative hobbies. Explore your particular passions in life and live them. Someone else cannot be made responsible for fulfilling your needs. Let go of the negative aspects in your lifestyle and relationship that hold you back, such as any compulsive or self-destructive elements.

Although it may be tempting to skip this section and get right down to the sexual techniques explained later in this book, make a vow to start at the beginning – by looking after yourself. All the time you spend nurturing yourself will ultimately enrich your relationship as well. You will have so much more to bring to your lover. The fuller you are, the more fulfilment you will find together. To bring bliss into your relationship, you can learn here how to experience this heightened state independently.

Then both of you can prioritize those aspects of your relationship that bring you nearer to joy and bliss, and enjoy it in abundance.

This Step shows you four Tantric principles with exercises that you can use now to release tension, and teaches you the Tantric secret of how to still the mind and awaken the sexual energy that fires your passion.

Relax and recharge your body

Your body is the temple of your spirit. For sex to be sacred, treat your body as sacred too. Most of us identify more with our minds than our bodies, but for Tantric masters you can conjure bliss most easily through your body. Your body is the site of your experience, the location of your opening up to the world. It is in your body that you feel precious moments of ecstasy, which are reached through bodily expression.

Consider the following; try them out as your daily mantras.

Through my body, I can transform my consciousness. I can be free from identifying myself only with my thoughts.

Through my body, I feel grounded and connected with everything around me.

Through my body, I can be in the moment and feel present, not tied to the past or the future.

Through my body, I can express everything there is to express, and do everything there is to achieve.

My body is awesome; its design, its function, its capacities. It is beautiful as it is.

Tantra describes the universe as a magical filament spun from threads of energy. The universe is dazzling, luminous. You are a part of this same fabric. You too are composed of vibrating energy. Worship the universe manifested in your being; learn to love what you see in the mirror. Your body is perfect and as lovely as a flower.

Total relaxation technique

The most important way to look after yourself is by learning to relax completely, so that you let go of tension in your body. Relaxing is not a waste of time. In fact, you may find that when you do nothing for a change, some of your most creative ideas pop into your head.

You can do the following three relaxation exercises every day. If you're a busy person with a stressful lifestyle, try to spend twenty minutes each day in total relaxation – you can split this into two ten-minute sessions.

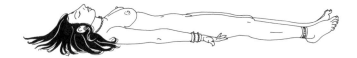

- Begin by lying down on the floor with your neck supported on a slim pillow or a book. As you stretch out, let your spine lengthen and bring up your knees. There's no need to press the small of your back flat into the floor – just let it relax naturally. Allow your head to drop back slightly, opening your jaw and letting your lips part. Throughout the exercise, keep your breathing natural and easy.
- Relax your body. With each breath, let go of muscular tightness in your body. Let your back settle into the floor. Let your shoulders release downwards into the floor, and focus your attention on allowing the holding in your neck to melt away. Release any tension in the small of your back. Imagine that your breathing releases any backache and heals any pain in your body. Let the soles of your feet sink into the earth.
- Now concentrate on widening your body. Let your hips spread out over the floor, taking up more space.
- Every time you breathe, mentally encourage every cell within your body to expand. Send your breath down to the bottom of your ribcage, letting your chest

expand more with each breath. Release any sense of holding or constriction, leaving more space for your heart to fill your chest. Let your shoulders spread out and take up more space. Let the healing energy of your breath dissolve muscular tension, stress and worry. Your healing breath can relieve tension and liberate your mind.

- As you breathe, close your eyes and visualize your inner self; deeply relax and allow this sense of you to be free to find its own state of rest.
- If your mind is distracted and busy, try to turn your eyes upwards. This reduces brain activity and promotes deep relaxation. Our bodies do this naturally when we sleep. You can also try this eye-turning technique during meditation or lovemaking, to still your mind if thoughts distract you.

Relax and chant

This exercise helps you relax deeply, using your voice to deepen your relaxation. The techniques here incorporate sound, so that your body sings as tension is released. The sound 'Om' expands your energy-body, or subtle inner energy *(see page 47)* and brings peace, clarity and bliss.

- Make yourself totally comfortable on a duvet or blanket folded on the floor, lying flat on your back with your arms by your sides. It helps if you focus on the heaviness of your body, letting the weight of it drop into the floor.
- When you feel relaxed, observe the rise and fall of your abdomen as you breathe in and out. Notice how your breathing slows down as you observe it.
- Allow your breathing to fall into a calm, easy rhythm. Let any muscular tension in your ribcage and abdomen melt away as each breath is expelled.
- Relax all the parts of your body, slowly moving from

the tips of your toes, through your ankles, calves, knees and thighs. With each breath direct your awareness to that area of your body, allowing yourself to relax more deeply with each out-breath.

- Focus your attention on your buttocks, relaxing them on the out-breath, and let your pelvis sink deeply into the floor. As you relax your pelvis and abdomen, say a long, drawn-out 'Ah'. Do this for several deeply relaxing exhalations. As you make the sound of 'Ah', let the vibrations from your chest spread through your pelvis to the rest of your body and down your legs. 'Ah' is a sound of openness – open yourself with every vocalization.

- When your lower body feels relaxed and energized, move your attention to your fingertips. Spend a few breaths relaxing your fingertips before moving through your hands, wrists, forearms, upper arms and shoulders. Allow your shoulders to relax more deeply with every out-breath, and let your spine sink into the duvet or blanket underneath.

- As you focus on your upper chest, draw your breath

into the area of your heart. As you release the breath, release an audible 'Oh' sound, letting the sound vibrations travel through your torso and down your arms.

- After several minutes breathing and chanting 'Oh', relax your neck, jaw and face. Spend the next few breaths relaxing your facial muscles, moving upwards towards the temples and to the top of your head. As you exhale, hum 'Mm', and allow the vibrations to resonate through your whole head. Do this for a few minutes.

- Now focus on your whole body fully relaxing. Combine the sounds 'Ah', 'Oh' and 'Mm' into the Sanskrit word for the sound of the universe: Om. As you exhale, chant 'Om', and let the vibrations spread throughout your whole body. Lie in a deep state of relaxation. Imagine every out-breath emanating from your vibrating body and into the endless space around you. Find repose and refreshment as you rest in this tranquil spaciousness.

Bring in the sun

The sun is a traditional Tantric symbol for the belly. In this exercise, you energize your belly through visualizing the warmth of the sun. This helps to release tension around the pelvis, freeing up your sexual energy.

Unfortunately, Western culture regards flat bellies as a sign of sexiness; however, in Tantra this muscular tightness is interpreted as a sign of sexual defence. Muscular tension is also a sign of stress – holding negative feelings in the area of your navel blocks the flow of energy through your body, producing further emotional and sexual disharmony. When your belly is hard and armoured as a result of anger or fear, it prevents your body from responding freely to the fire of your sexual passion, which also blocks the connection between your sexual desire and your loving emotions.

You can also benefit from this visualization exercise if your belly is loose and flabby, which in Tantra is a symptom of neglect of your vital and sexual energy. By imagining that you are absorbing sustenance from the sun, you refuel with energy. In allowing the energy to fill you up, you encourage your belly to charge your life force, a resource for your whole body.

To begin, stretch out on the floor with your knees up, relaxing your spine as described in the Total relaxation exercise above.

- Become aware of your breathing. Breathe in and out of your mouth for some minutes, then relax and let your breath breathe itself.
- Now focus on slowing down your breathing, and let each breath sink into your belly. Let your belly soften. Allow your belly to rise with every inhalation, and fall with every exhalation. Keep breathing into your belly until you lose track of time. Become your breathing.
- After a while, draw down your breath from your lungs into your abdomen. At the end of every inhalation, briefly pause, holding your breath, and visualize an imaginary sun resting in your belly. As you continue to draw in the rays of the sun, let your belly absorb its light and heat, and allow your abdominal

muscles to soften. Encourage the sun's warmth to spread throughout your body and limbs. Your whole being feels languid and completely relaxed, just as it does when you are sunbathing. Luxuriate in the goodness of the sun.

Heal your body

Many of us have stress patterns in our bodies as a result of old injuries, shock and illness. However, day-to-day pressures also imprint stress in our tissues. This creates a pattern of stress that means we habitually react to challenges in a harmful way; our stress causes energy to become constricted in the body, which in turn creates physical tension and pain. Chronic tension produces common problems such as headaches, insomnia, anxiety and irritability. Tension can lead to a host of other problems, which may often prove unresponsive to medication.

Some couples use sex as a way of releasing tension, but this is a waste of the potential riches that good lovemaking can bring you. Conversely, too much stress may put you off sex all together. If you are carrying tension in your body, you need to release it before sex rather than during sex. You can't hope to access sexual bliss if you are using sex to deal with the build-up of stress in your system. If you're relaxed, balanced and harmonized before making love, you will get so much more out of the experience. Below are two Tantric techniques to get you started – the Healing breath exercise below, where you direct your breath to specific areas of your body; and the Light laundry in which you use visualized light to wash away the stress of the day.

Healing breath

This technique uses breathing techniques for healing, and helps you to feel compassion towards yourself by treating your body with appreciation. To begin, lie down, relax and breathe as described in the Total relaxation exercise *(see page 6)*.

- Breathe deeply for a few minutes. Then focus on the breath breathing itself as described in the previous exercise, Bring in the sun *(see page 12)*. Evoke a sense of marvel at your body.
- Feel thankful for your body, and appreciate it for the support it gives you in achieving your daily demands. Feel compassionate toward its aches and weaknesses.
- As you breathe, imagine that you are sending healing breath directly into any part of your body that feels tense or uncomfortable. Send healing energy into any part that is in pain.
- Allow this healing breath to radiate through your body for several moments. Notice how your body expands with the loving concern of your attention.

The light laundry

This exercise uses the Tantric image of radiant light to literally wash out stress patterns held in your body. Light is a form of vital energy that is visualized to purify your mind and body. It takes only a few minutes every day to practise this exercise, and it's a good way to deal with the day's accumulated stress when you come home from work. You can also use this technique as an energy-boost at the beginning of the day, or perhaps before lovemaking.

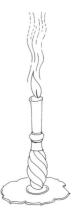

You can prepare for this meditation by turning off any artificial lights and filling the room with candles. Otherwise, visualize the light in your mind's eye.

- Lie down, sit cross-legged on the floor, or in a chair with a straight back to allow energy to move freely up and down your spine. If you are sitting, rest your hands on your knees, with palms upturned to receive energy.
- Focus on your breathing. As you observe the fall and rise of your breath, imagine that your whole body is illuminated with light. With every in-breath, absorb more light into your body.

17

- Imagine that light is flooding every tissue of your body, throwing a spotlight on any darkness, tension or pain. See this healing light fill your shoulders, head and spine, your heart, chest and pelvis. Let the clarity of the light rest on any tension. As you breathe out, release this holding pattern of energy.
- Encourage the light to become more intense throughout your body, and feel it hum with vitality as your body is radiated. Let the light illuminate every cell and pore.
- Visualize the light pouring through you, like a pure, fresh rain drenching you, washing your body from your toes up to your head.
- Spend several minutes resting in the luminosity as your body fills with light. Let the light dissolve any shadows within. You are clear as a crystal, full of light yet opaque. You are made entirely of light. Imagine that everything in the universe is composed of light, and that light surrounds you everywhere.

Get supple

Look after your body's primary needs. Your body needs to move, to stretch and work out. For good sex it helps if you are supple, limber and fit – but you don't need to become obsessed about working out in the gym in order to achieve this. The simplest way to improve your energy is to become more physically active. If you're chronically tired, remember that expending energy usually gives you more energy. Any exercise that you enjoy will boost your metabolism and improve your natural energy.

Pilates is superb, because it combines working the muscles of the pelvic floor with stretches and breathing; in Tantra, it is essential to work on your breathing and improve your pelvic floor muscles to enhance your ability to feel erotic pleasure during sex *(see page 162)*. Yoga is a beautifully balanced combination of stretching, breathing, relaxation and inner focus *(see the yoga exercises on page 25)*.

You will also benefit from the tension release that regular exercise brings. The upper body, the small of the

19

back and the pelvis are common tension sites, so these areas will respond well to stretches. Swimming improves your lung capacity and releases tension around the upper body. You can also free up your pelvis with oriental belly dancing, or Latin dance such as salsa. These styles of dance are great for making you feel sexually confident, playful and flirtatious *(see page 104 for dance techniques)*. Remember that Tantric sex is about relaxing into your sensuality and your erotic relationship. To achieve this, you need to deal with the tension in your body before lovemaking, rather than rely on your partner to give you release through orgasm. Your partner is probably just as stressed as you are.

Exercise should be a pleasure rather than a chore; listen to your body and take note of what you enjoy, rather than forcing yourself to work out for the sake of it. It is important to think about what your body responds to, and decide what you can do to feel enlivened. If you decide to devise your own workout, start with gentle stretches, but remember to breathe deeply as you stretch. Deep breathing nourishes your body with oxygen. This cleanses and detoxifies your muscles, helping them relax and preventing injury.

Dancing for sexual energy

Dance styles such as tango have long been described as akin to horizontal sex. In this exercise, you treat yourself and your partner to a session of sensual dancing at home. Without anyone watching you, you can forget your

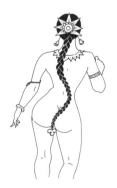

mutual inhibitions and enjoy the mutual buzz of dancing together. Dancing lessens your self-consciousness because the music encourages you to respond instinctively. If you find this fun, enjoy a regular dance session in which you play all your favourite music.

- With your lover, take turns playing music you love, sometimes dancing for their delectation while they watch, sometimes dancing together.
- As you get absorbed in the dance, abandon yourself to expressing the music through your body. Free yourself. Don't think about what you are doing or how you look. Let the music dance you.
- Explore the various dynamics between you, sometimes creatively sparking off each other, harmonizing, complementing, finding your own space, melting together.
- Explore different rhythms – staccato, lyrical or wild. Try periods of stillness when it feels appropriate, when you just stop and sense your being vibrating with the rhythm of your dancing and the grace of your movements.

Eating for energy and sensuality

Self-nourishment is a primary need – food is literally used to nurture. If you've withheld food from yourself you may wish to relearn how to feed yourself with abundant good food. Your body needs healthy foods: a basic nutritious diet includes whole grains, legumes, pulses, lean meat, fish, and plenty of fresh fruits and vegetables to feed your body with essential vitamins and minerals. A nutritious diet and regular meals also promote a sustained release of energy throughout the day. This helps avoid the blood-sugar highs and lows that can lead to cravings for carbohydrates and foods high in fat and sugar that are so common in our fast-food culture.

Tantra is not an ascetic path that recommends self-denial in any way. Indian practitioners used alcohol and cannabis as part of their rites, as well as meat and fish, which are normally prohibited for Hindus. It's not what you eat that has erotic potential, but how you eat it. As a path of sensual pleasure, Tantra emphasizes the natural sensuality of preparing and eating good food. Eating is also a ritual celebration of togetherness, which is communally expressed at mealtimes in Mediterranean and Eastern cultures. You can make any small meal into an occasion for expressing your love.

- Sexiness is about paying attention to what your lover enjoys eating, and taking time and care in its purchase and preparation. Don't forget the table setting, with candles and flowers, and do dress (or undress) for dinner.
- Choose ingredients that stimulate your palate, balancing tastes so that different flavours complement each other. Consider the texture and visual qualities of the food, as well as the taste.
- Serve your partner in an attentive manner, making sure that everything needed is available. There's nothing

> sexier than an ardent waiter offering you tasty titbits.
>
> - If you want to use food as part of your lovemaking, a fun idea is to prepare soft foods that can be eaten off your lover's body – avocados, bananas, strawberries and mangoes have the ideal consistency. Chocolate has aphrodisiac properties and can be melted, painted on and then licked off.

The yoga of tantra

Yoga postures encourage the release of any tension held around the hips, pelvis and shoulders. Yoga was used by Indian Tantrics to develop physical suppleness and breath control. The art of yoga is centred on your breathing, and your energy is centred, or grounded, down in your sacrum. Yogic breathing builds your energy in your pelvis and then directs it from your hips and upwards through your body.

Warm up

These warm-up exercises stretch and loosen the hips, pelvis and inner thighs. Begin by sitting comfortably on the floor with your legs crossed loosely and your back straight.

- Concentrate on your breathing, directing your in-breaths into your abdomen. As you inhale through your mouth, relax your jaw. Relax your throat and open your lungs as the air moves down. Release your ribcage so that your lungs can open fully. Relax the muscles under your ribcage, opening the diaphragm and letting the air fill your belly. Keep your belly soft and relaxed.
- As you breathe, release your lower back. Do this by moving your waist from side to side, letting the rhythm move upwards so that your upper back, shoulders and neck are gently undulating. Let your back uncoil, and keep moving your shoulders from side to side to release tension. Let your neck join in. Once your back feels more flexible, spend a little time releasing your neck. If you don't suffer from neck pain, you can roll

your head around your neck slowly and gently. Let it fall backwards as far as is comfortable.

- Now lie on your back with your buttocks touching the wall and your legs straight up, resting on the wall. Settle your spine into the floor. When you are comfortable, let your legs slide open, and exhale as you hold the stretch. Slowly slide your legs together again as you inhale. Do this several times.

- Sit comfortably upright, with your legs opened out in a 'v' shape. If you are practising with your partner and are quite flexible, you can sit on the floor facing each other with your feet touching. Bend forward for a few minutes, loosening up the muscles and tendons before reaching forward to hold your partner's hands. Using the weight of your partner as a gentle counter-balance, let your upper bodies rotate in a circle together. Be very careful not to pull too hard and strain a muscle. If you are practising alone, bend forward and place your palms on the floor between your legs. Allow your body to rotate as you gently push against your hands.

27

Squat!

Practising squatting can give you more stamina during active lovemaking postures where the woman is on top. Squatting releases tension and opens out your pelvis, stretching the muscles around the hips.

- Move into a standing position with your feet hip-width apart. Keep your feet parallel as you bend your knees and sit on your haunches, moving into a squatting position. Your weight should be on your heels, with your buttocks hovering just above the floor; be careful not to strain the tendons in your ankles. Sit for

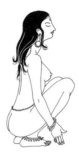

several minutes at least, breathing into your lower abdomen. With each out-breath, focus on relaxing all the muscles around your hips and pelvis. Let your pelvis open more with each inhalation, and release even more tension with every exhalation.

Swing your hips

- Stand up and place your hands on your hips. Circle your hips as if you were tracing a hoop, easing all your muscles as you move in a gradually wider circle. Inhale for half a circle, and exhale for the other half. Pause with each in-breath, just before you begin each half-circle.

- Try describing a horizontal figure of eight with your hips.

Release your upper back

Repeat the squat position described above.

- As your hips and ankles ease into the posture, relax the top half of your body, letting your head hang forward and your arms drop loosely between your knees. Let all the tension you are carrying around your shoulders and upper back drop away.

Release your shoulders

- If your shoulders still feel tense, slowly bring your upper body into a standing position again. Then bring both arms behind your back, holding the palm of one hand in the other, with your arms straight. As you bend forward your arms will fall away from your body.
- Remain in this position, bent over with clasped hands, relaxing the tension around your shoulders as you breathe.

Corpse pose

In yoga, the corpse is the traditional name for the relaxation pose used at the end or beginning of a sequence of postures. In lovemaking, the corpse posture is when the man lies underneath his partner.

- Lie flat on your back on the floor, with arms relaxed by your side and your palms facing upwards. To lengthen your back and straighten your spine, start with your knees bent upward and focus on relaxing the small of your back, settling it into the floor. When your back is comfortable, lengthen your neck by drawing your chin more toward your chest.

- With your next few breaths, straighten your legs along the floor, with your feet slightly apart.
- Spend several minutes relaxing. Concentrate on the breath moving through your airways, filling your throat, sternum and ribcage, and releasing all the muscular tension as you breathe out.

Make a bridge

Remain lying down for the four final postures.

- With your knees bent upward and your arms along your side, slowly lift up your hips as you breathe out, letting the breath go right down into the centre of your pelvis. With each out-breath unfurl your back, lifting it from the floor. Leave your neck extended and in contact with the floor, but lift up your back right up

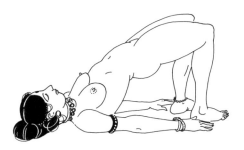

to your shoulders. With every out-breath, release any tension you can feel. Think that you are offering your body to the universe; your body is a bridge for your energy to move outward.

- Let your back relax and move slowly downwards. Begin with your shoulders, then release your back, hips and buttocks, so you return to the corpse pose.

Release

- Bring up your knees, keeping the soles of your feet resting flat on the floor and the small of your back snuggling into the floor. Place your hands, palms down, over your heart area, and focus on breathing into your heart. Let your arms fully relax, with your elbows resting on the floor. Your fingertips should touch each other.

The butterfly

The butterfly describes the action of your bent knees, which move together and apart like butterfly wings. This exercise opens your pelvis to sexual energy.

- Open your knees to each side as you breathe in, taking the breath all the way down to your pelvis. Exhale, and relax into the posture with a feeling of surrender.
- Take another breath in and, as you exhale, press your feet together and down into the floor in order to bring your knees back to the upright position. If this is at all uncomfortable for your back or hips, support each thigh with cushions.
- When you have familiarized yourself with this 'out-in' movement of your legs, switch your attention back to the rise and fall of your abdomen with your breath.

33

Surrender

The posture of surrender focuses your attention on the movement of sexual energy by drawing your breath in and out through your genitals.

- Lie on your back, with your arms out to the side and your palms facing upwards. Let your knees drop to the floor on either side, placing the soles of both feet together. If you are not very flexible, don't bend your knees quite so much, but leave the soles of your feet together. As you inhale, imagine that you are drawing in energy through your genitals and the base of your spine; in your mind's eye, see it climbing up your spine and resting at the crown of your head as you finish inhaling. As you exhale, visualize that your breath drops back down to your genitals and streams out through them.

To finish

Repeat the corpse pose *(see page 30)*, and relax for at least five minutes.

Get a head start: meditation

Most meditation practices start with paying attention to your breath. Breath is the source of our vitality; it is how we live. In Sanskrit, the word for 'breath' means 'spirit'. Breathing deeply also stimulates your unique energy-body, the internal, subtle energy that is stimulated through Tantric practice *(see page 48)*.

The best posture to meditate in is 'easy pose', which helps to keep your back upright while sitting for long periods. Sit with your feet crossed at the level of the calves so that each foot is under the opposite knee.

How to breathe

This breath meditation helps relax your body, and bring your mind to the present – it is this quality of presence that makes sex ecstatic, when you focus on sensation and feel the exchange of love between you and your partner. By practising breath meditation, you can let energy radiate from your breath and animate your body; when you make love, you can feel intensely in the moment.

- Sit with your legs crossed loosely in easy pose, with one leg in front of the other. Sense your relaxed body. Summon up a sense of wonder at the miracle of being alive. Breathe fully, right down into your abdomen. This expands your lung capacity, and slows down the rate of your breathing.
- Pause for a moment or two before you inhale, and before exhaling. Then lengthen the holding-in stage of your breath, as well as the exhalation, so that you inhale for a count of one, hold for four, and exhale for two.
- Pay attention to each out-breath and fully relax on each one. Let go. The in-breath will take care of itself.

When you have mastered this technique, you can use it in all the meditations in this book. You can progress your practice by focusing your inner eye on visualization to encourage the natural movement of energy through your body *(see page 48)*.

Get centred

Grounding, or centring yourself is a basic technique that deepens your sense of being; it helps you to feel connected and complete. When you are with your partner you can be self-contained, but also open to share your energy; in Tantra, this is a building block for intimacy. Grounding is also recommended as a relaxation technique after dynamic freestyle dancing; learn how to move from a state of high energy into this blissful, centring meditation.

- Stand with your feet hip-distance apart and your knees slightly bent, with your back straight. This helps align your spine so that energy can move through your body more easily.
- Close your eyes and focus your attention on your breathing. Be aware of your inhalation and exhalation, without trying to control it. Observe it for a few minutes. You will probably notice that your breathing calms down and becomes longer and more even just by paying attention to it.

- Inhale, and imagine that your breath is travelling down to the base of your spine, right to your tailbone. As you exhale, imagine it moving back up your spine to exit through your lungs.
- Imagine that you are a new tree growing roots. Visualize these conduits of energy reaching deep down into the earth. As you breathe in and out, your roots are expanding, growing, reaching through the layers of earth. With each out-breath, let your roots penetrate even deeper as if they are striving to touch the centre of the earth. This symbolizes your connection to the earth as a source of energy. Feel this vital energy pouring into you through your roots.
- As you continue to breathe, draw this nurturing source of life and energy up your spine so that it can permeate your body. Keep breathing and drawing this energy up through the soles of your feet, creating a sense of solidity and groundedness.
- Then draw that energy up into your pelvis and torso and into your lungs and chest, allowing your lungs to expand fully.

- Breathe in, drawing that energy into the centre of your chest, in the area of your heart. Feel your heart expand with your breath, and fill with energy for life and love.
- Fill your head with energy. Imagine that you are growing branches of energy that touch the sky from the crown of your head. Feel these vital conduits reach into space, the realm of the infinite and of the spirit.
- Feel a sense of infinite possibility. Mentally bring down this sense of expansion and spaciousness through the branches in the sky and into the crown at the top of your head. Then bring this sensation into your chest; let your heart feel soothed. Imagine the spaciousness of the heavens mingling with the grounding energy of the earth in your heart. See your heart as the centre of convergence whose roots connect with the earth, and whose branches connect with heaven. You are a bridge between the two.

Ground yourself in nature

Start with this simple visualization exercise to learn how to take in energy from outside in order to balance your own internal energy. When you feel more connected to the earth – literally grounded – you are better able to remain yourself while in the energy field of others. This helps you to maintain your self-esteem and internal balance.

- Imagine yourself in a favourite landscape. If you feel most at peace in woodlands, mountains or meadows, imagine yourself there. In your mind's eye, picture the landscape, the rocks and trees, foliage and flowers. If the seaside gives you most energy, visualize yourself on a shore, feet in the sand, gazing at the ocean. Go inside yourself and commune with nature. Feel connected and nourished by what is around you.
- Relax and feel the environment holding you. You are resting in the waves of the ocean, or the leaves and grasses all around you.

- Absorb the goodness and strength of nature. Imagine that everything around you gives you energy and light.

On finding stillness

Meditation masters say that you don't need to do anything in order to find stillness; you simply cease your activity to stop doing and start being. Yet it can be difficult to find stillness, because we need to learn to quiet the incessant chatter of our minds. Our minds are often charged and over-stimulated; our normal state of mind is restless, chaotic and overrun with myriad thoughts that push and pull us in different directions.

Sages hold that thoughts are a distraction from your true self, and this sense of authenticity can only emerge in the gaps between thoughts – the time when your thoughts are not there to claim your attention. This is the authentic self, an inherent quality of presence that is not defined by what we do or our identity labels. It is a quality of consciousness that is open, responsive and vibrant.

When you let go of your mind, you also let go of your

41

ego. Your ego is the idea you have of yourself that is made up of your thoughts about yourself. These are usually negative thoughts and create what psychologists call a 'false' self – an idea of yourself that is not based on the reality of who you are. Your authentic nature is a state of being experienced in meditation, in lovemaking, in peak experiences where you feel moved into a realm of ecstasy. These are all times when you transcend a limited idea of who you are and what you are capable of experiencing. By shifting your focus to clear and still your mind, you make way for your own ecstasy.

Shift your focus, clear your mind

The most important thing to do in order to experience a different state of being is to stop thinking and allow yourself to be entirely in the present, not the future. You can transform your experience of anything by shifting the focus of your attention. By mastering this technique, you get more out of everything that you do. During

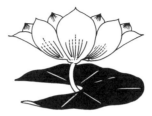

lovemaking, you can experience more intense pleasure by simply choosing to focus on your pleasure.

- You can use any mundane activity as a meditation. While you're walking to work, focus on enjoying every step of the way. Rather than mentally plan all the things you have to do, absorb the detail of what's around you.
- At home, apply this approach to the tasks you loathe. Enjoy the sensory experience of washing up; slow it down, watch the bubbles, trace the water.
- Choose one focus for your mind. Channel all its powers into a single point, such as gazing at a flower. Let looking absorb all your mental energy. Keep

practising this until you can hold the object in your mind's eye, unwavering, for at least five minutes. When you have mastered this you can try sitting in meditation in front of a flickering candle flame, or just focus on the slow inhalation and exhalation of your breath.

Witness your thoughts

Sitting quietly and watching your thoughts is the first step to developing some degree of detachment from them. It is your thoughts that create a screen composed of preconceptions, judgments and interpretations that hamper relating. The first step to disengaging from the ceaseless activity of your mind is to become a witness to the process.

• Let any thoughts that enter your mind come and go without captivating your interest. Don't struggle to control your thoughts; the best way to deal with them is to keep bringing your awareness back to your breathing. Breathe in, feeling the air fill your chest, and push your abdomen gently outwards. Hold the breath without any tension in your body, and then gently release the air.

- You will notice how often your mind pulls away from focusing on a simple act with all sorts of distractions. Don't try to control your mind. The art of meditation is in letting go of thoughts, rather than trying to force your mind to be somewhere. Just observe your thoughts.

Meditation and sex

Tantra provides the perfect method and the motivation for keeping you in the moment: sex. Sex is one of the few moments in everyday life when we are able to suspend our thoughts; this is the sort of thought-gap that we aim for in meditation.

For most people sex provides one of the few peak experiences in life. Tantra holds that life can be like this all the time, if you learn to transform your consciousness. Life is really a vibrant, energizing, delicious stream of energy, if you can just let go of what you think life is all about and who you think you are. Letting go of preconceived ideas will automatically uncover a more authentic way of being.

Meditate on your sexual energy

After a relaxing bath, light a candle in front of a mirror. Gaze at your naked body in the mirror. Appreciate the beauty of your form. Then close your eyes and go inward.

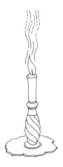

- Enjoy the sensuality of your body. You are your sexuality.
- Let eroticism spread throughout your whole being. Draw your breath down into your pelvis, and then into your sexual organs. Sense them warm and alive, suffusing your body with sexual energy. Let a sensual glow radiate from your body.
- Enjoy being alive. Enjoy being sexy. Appreciate the sense of wellbeing that awakening your sexual nature allows you. Celebrate the presence of erotic energy – it is not only in you, it is all around you. Plug into it and let your erotic nature explode.
- Melt into sexual bliss.

Get a sexual energy-body

The sexual energy-body is part of the subtle body inside us that we can feel but not touch. The more you become aware of your own energy-body, the more you improve your wellbeing and enhance your sexual satisfaction. You also improve your ability to connect with your partner and sustain that connection. Working with Tantric techniques helps you to open your heart to more love, becoming more aware of the importance of love as well as the sacredness of life. One of the best by-products of awakening your internal energy-body is achieving a state of dynamic meditation; this is when you feel vibrant, but amazingly relaxed.

Body therapists have discovered that the movement of energy through the body clears physical tension produced by holding your body tight, and promotes healthy function. Therapists release this by encouraging physical movement and paying attention to the streaming of energy in the body. This is close to the way Tantra views the relationship between the subtle energy-body and our physical body. Your natural state of energy is one of constant flow.

Feeling your unique energy-body

This meditation helps you sense and connect with the vitality of your inner body of energy.

- Close your eyes to focus on sensing your body from within. Let your body revel in its vitality. Focus your awareness on your pelvis, feeling it radiating energy. Let the energy spread from your pelvis into your chest and heart area. Feel the energy in your head, arms and hands. Let the energy spread from your hips and buttocks down into your legs and feet.
- Relax into your body more deeply. Sense how this energy pervades your heart, your lungs, your muscles and every tissue of your body. Focus on the sensation inside your body.
- Feel that every cell of your body is full of vitality, vibrating with energy. Focus all your attention on this.
- Let go of the form of your body. Pay attention to the feel of this energy, visualizing the finely vibrating atoms and molecules. Feel how your body is made up of energy; you are just a small part of a vast energy field.
- Sense how the subtle energy field that makes up the universe permeates you. Let it course throughout your whole body.

Awaken your inner fire

This meditation helps you to connect with your natural erotic energy.

- Lie down comfortably, allowing your whole body to relax. Focus on your gentle breathing.
- Feel your sexual energy emanating from your pelvis. Sense it penetrating your whole body. Revel in the sensuality of your body.
- Imagine an intense, inner heat at the core of your being. Visualize this as red fire permeating your body.

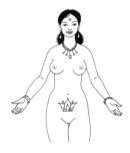

Let your sexual energy enliven you – don't think, feel it: feel your sexual being. Embrace that sexual power.

As you go about your daily life, allow this sexual energy to be in your awareness. Don't cut off from it, judging it inappropriate, embarrassing or distracting. Sexuality is your true nature.

Allow it to colour your interactions with warmth, passion and sexual presence.

The chakra energy map

The energy-body has been documented over thousands of years. The body's energy system is considered to be a microcosm of the universe. In this model, there is usually a central conduit of energy from the base of the spine to the crown of the head, fed by two main channels on either side and a network of subsidiary arteries. Along

51

the main channels are areas where the energy gathers and seems particularly intense. These are described as chakras, or wheels of energy. There are seven principle chakras, and myriad minor chakra points.

At the crown of the head is the seventh chakra, where mind and body, heart and soul are unified. Tantric practitioners describe this unification symbolically as the lovemaking of the divine goddess and her consort, whose sexual satisfaction creates a cosmic state of bliss and connectedness.

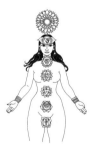

Give yourself pleasure

Sensual pleasure is vital for your wellbeing. It nurtures your body and opens you to sexual experience, enhancing your life. You need pleasure as an affirmation of your right to happiness and joy. Touch and nurturing are healing. The need for touch is crucial for survival and development – so touch yourself.

You need pleasure in your life, so learn to prioritize pleasure. Think about what gives you pleasure; you might want to write down all the things you enjoy doing, and then think about how much (or how little) time you actually spend doing those things.

It's important to make more time for yourself. You can nourish yourself and your loved ones with touch, with food, with sleep, with sex. By focusing more on the sensual pleasure provided through sensory contact, you will get more from it. Demonstrating your love and affection creates an atmosphere of love, which nourishes you too. Being demonstrative affirms your own positive feelings.

Sensuous touch

Touch is a vital means of opening to pleasure. Through touch, you can reacquaint your body with subtle sensation. Slow and gentle touch allows you to relax into the sensation more fully. Touch each other gracefully, with gentleness. Have a session in which you spend time exploring the surfaces of each other's body, enjoying the shapes, textures and smells of your partner's flesh.

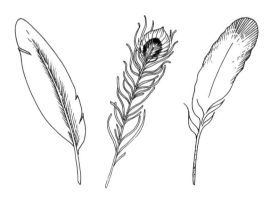

- When you touch your lover, keep your touch light. Imagine that you are tracing exquisite designs on your lover's skin.
- Think of softer, slower ways of touching your partner; this way sensuality arises naturally and won't feel contrived.

Try using your fingertips, your fingernails or a feather to touch. Touch through silk, or massage with textured food like avocado puree or natural yoghurt.

Massage

Massage is about feeling good in your body, releasing tension, relaxing, receiving and surrendering to love. You can practise self-massage, or enjoy giving and receiving massage with your partner. It's a good way to nurture each other, to feel cared for and looked after. Knotted muscles can be kneaded out, aches and stiffness released, worries stroked away and skin stimulated. By relaxing your partner through massage, you prepare him or her to receive your love and absorb your tenderness.

If your partner is going through a phase of not feeling sexually alive or responsive, massage maintains the physical contact that you associate with lovemaking. When you are having a difficult time sexually, massage helps you keep touching in a safe, non-pressurized way. All sex therapists suggest opting for non-genital touch and massage whenever your lovemaking is not working for one or both of you, and you need to work towards a new style of lovemaking. Your partner will relax more if massage is not set up as a prelude to sex, but something to enjoy for its own sake. Massage is about giving, without expectation of receiving – and receiving without feeling that you have to reciprocate. Sex, however, assumes that you will be responsive, and if your partner is not in the mood they will experience your desire as a pressure to satisfy your needs.

Sensual massage technique

There are a few golden rules for massage:

1 Keep the room warm. You may like to cover the parts of the body that you are not massaging with a warm towel.
2 Place a few drops of massage oil in your palms and rub them together to warm the oil before you apply it.

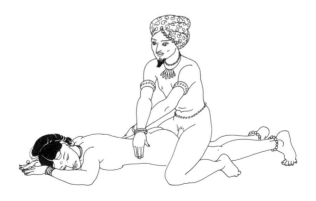

3 Keep one hand on your partner at all times; it's distracting if your partner doesn't feel your touch and then you suddenly place your hands on their body.

- Start with your partner lying on their front and work on the area just above the buttocks. Use long strokes, sweeping from the base of the spine (on either side of the vertebrae rather than directly on the bones) up to the shoulders – use one hand on each side of the spine.
- Knead the buttocks and work up along the spine.
- Pay attention to releasing the muscles around the shoulder blades, starting on either side of the spine and moving around the side of the shoulder blade and then towards the shoulder joints. You may want to use both hands to knead the area above the shoulder blade, working first on one side, then on the other side of the body.
- Massage along the side of the neck vertebra and into the base of the neck.
- Once you have relaxed your partner's body, you can start exploring different strokes, varying the rhythm

and depth of pressure. Be careful not to hurt your partner at any stage, and always stop immediately if he or she feels uncomfortable. Ask for feedback throughout, so you can respond to your partner's needs.

Self-pleasuring

Self-pleasuring is the key to taking responsibility for your own sexual satisfaction. Through self-exploration, you can learn about your own unique sexual response and focus on the subtleties of your own erotic pleasure. You can jettison old habitual ways of stimulating yourself if they aren't particularly pleasurable, and discover new sensations. When you learn how to extend your erotic pleasure, you can share this knowledge with your sexual partner. Through experiencing yourself as pleasure, you can later include your partner in your pleasure.

As you pleasure yourself, allow your feelings to arise without judging yourself. Appreciate your positive qualities, and accept those that you know you struggle with (shyness, embarrassment or shame, for example). If you can achieve this, you will be able to reconnect with your passion for yourself, others and your life.

Make love to yourself

In order to connect with your sexual energy, make love to yourself. Set the scene by making sure the room is warm and put on some sensual, inviting music. Light some candles and a stick of incense, and crush some flower petals into a bowl of water. Then anoint your body with talcum powder or oil, appreciating the soft sensation of your flesh.

- Sit comfortably as you start to anoint your skin with massage oil, or use talc if you don't want to get too oily. Enjoy the feel of your body under your hands as well as the way your hands feel to your body.
- Explore your body as if you were your own lover. Treat the experience like a meditation, relaxing into it.

Take your time, experimenting with different touches. Stroke yourself with a feather, your hands, talcum powder or massage oil. Discover the sensitivity of different areas, paying particular attention to those you habitually neglect. Enter fully into the experience of your own pleasure.

• After some time, focus on your genitals. Women: Oil your genitals all over – your inner thighs, vulva, inner lips and your anus. Explore the delicate skin on the inside of your thighs, perhaps stroking your breasts at the same time. Touch your inner and outer lips, and all the surfaces of your genitals. Play around the clitoris, using a finger on each side to rub up and down. Circle around the clitoris, or gently rub the hood over the clitoris. Take plenty of time in order to find out what feels delicious, and to immerse yourself in your own pleasure.

• Men: Try different strokes and ways of touching yourself. Use your hand to hold your penis with your thumb facing up or down. Use one hand or two to cradle your genitals. Use your hand to make a ring around your penis. Roll your penis between your hands, or use rhythmic, stroking movements up and down its length. Cradle your scrotum, and rub or gently squeeze. Rub the fleshy mound behind your scrotum, which is the external prostate spot. As you get aroused by stroking your genitals, you may like to explore the perineum (the area between the scrotum and anus) and the anus, as this area becomes more pleasurable when engorged with blood.

- As you get really aroused, encourage a sensation of fine sexual energy to stream upwards from your genitals, warming your body.
- Bring the self-pleasuring to a close by bringing one hand to rest over your pubic mound, and the other between your breasts, at your heart. Let sexual pleasure fill your heart.
- Afterwards, relax in a luxurious warm bath.

Get connected: finding intimacy

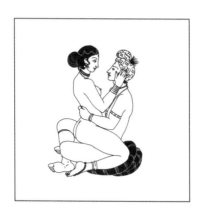

Connection is a fundamental need. The drive for connection is the reason why we are all in relationship with others. Couples who are more connected feel happier in their relationship and their lives in general. They communicate well, and demonstrate how much they care about each other's priorities in life.

A sense of connection is fundamental to Tantric sex. It covers many levels: emotional, sexual, loving, sharing a sense of vision and acknowledging your deep bond as soul mates. Tantra encompasses all these aspects of a relationship, and its practice encourages you to unify your two individual selves into a single 'body' of energy. This body is composed of love.

When you have awakened your own energy *(see Step 1, pages 46–52)* you can direct it toward another in love. In the same way that you care for yourself, you can take care of your lover. Rather than relate to one another on the basis of your personalities, learn to see your lover as an energy-body with whom you bond at heart level. Personality traits act as surface distraction, which get in the way of love energy. When we become

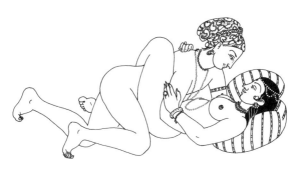

irritated with our beloved's traits, this creates additional blocks to intimacy. You can use your energy to create a bridge between the two of you, which will keep you clear of the obstacles that risk causing your relationship to founder.

Feeling connected helps you stay close to one another so that you no longer feel separate or alone. In experiencing togetherness, your true self emerges; you can enjoy your natural state of connectedness with others. When you care for yourself by meeting your inherent need to share, you heal your loneliness. You can express empathy for others and know how they feel.

Making an authentic connection

Honest communication is an indicator of a good relationship. If you don't feel understood, ask yourself if you really understand your partner. How can you expect your lover to know what you want if you don't have sufficient empathy to understand them? You may need to work harder at understanding their motivation before you can develop a deeper communication and connection in your sexual relationship.

For deep communication, you need to be in touch with the depths of your own life. Living authentically means finding your passion by expressing yourself creatively. Ask yourself whether you are living according to your authentic nature – are you doing what you love doing? Are you expressing what is deep inside you? Are you speaking your truth?

Speak your truth

Make communication real; don't fake it. You don't need to fake anything you don't feel. The key to real power is authenticity. You own your personal power when you take the risk of expressing your deepest truths. This expression may be an active decision to align yourself with your deeper nature. You can simply communicate your reality as it is, without pretence.

Use open communication to create harmony and purpose in your sexual relationship. This means speaking your truth and being heard, but remaining open and being willing to hear the truth of others. Look at the ways in which these truths are manifested in your life and love.

Surrender the need to control

Drop your defences and pretences. Frustration in a relationship can arise through attempting to impose your will or to make things happen. This creates a high level

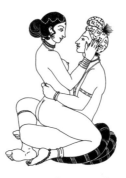

of tension. You may need to stop doing – to stop trying so hard – to make your relationship work in the way that you want. When you surrender any attempt at control and spend time being, rather than doing, you ultimately gain your personal power. Being too pushy creates rigidity, stress and suspicion. Being too passive creates a lack of focus and a tendency to escape daily life through daydreaming. Find your centre of balance and maintain it. Equally, don't do anything sexually that you don't want to do. Share your sexual secrets to defuse them. Deepen your trust.

Anger is often a sign of frustrated will. Let go of the frustration of attempting to impose your will. Experiment by not trying to push for your goal, or forcing yourself to carry on. Learn deep relaxation, and use meditation and yoga to let go of physical and mental rigidity *(see pages 6, 25)*. Nurture yourself and each other.

Noble speech

To heal emotional confusion it is essential to speak your truth. You need to communicate clearly what is important to you in your relationship so that your partner knows what your fundamental agenda is. For instance, if there are commitment problems in your relationship, you both need to be honest about your attitudes toward commitment.

While it is essential to hold onto your inner truth, Buddhists believe that it is important to consider the context of your speech before you speak. It is not okay to say what you want to say, regardless of the feelings of the listener or the consequences of your words. Buddhist precepts are fundamental to courteous, harmonious interaction.

Your words should be gentle and courteous, and
go straight to the heart.

Your speech should be aimed at spreading
harmony, uniting what is divided.

What you say should be said in the right context
and at an appropriate moment.

Unless you can contribute something
constructive, maintain a noble silence.

Don't repeat in one place what you have heard in
another; avoid gossip, slander and harsh language.

Communicate your kind intentions rather than
anger.

Avoid putting others down; remind yourself of
your limitations before rushing to criticize
another.

Don't try to impose your will on others. Do not hurt them intentionally, or dishonour them.

Speak about what you know, and admit it if you don't know. Speak in accordance with facts, rather than your beliefs.

Be honest about any mistakes that you have made.

You need to remain open and loving with others rather than relate solely according to your own ego-centred needs. The Buddhist moral code is steeped in morality because of their belief in karma. Karma focuses on the relation of cause and effect – meaning that everything you do has a ripple effect on those around you. When you become aware of the serious effects of your smallest actions, you can then take responsibility for the consequences of all your actions. Whatever it is you are doing, make sure that you do no harm to other living beings.

Loving with attitude

Love is the heart of your relationship. Yet so many of us are emotionally wounded that our whole society seems afflicted by a deficit of love. Healing begins with attitude and intent. To help heal your heart, contemplate the following.

My heart energy is activated when I connect with others, my environment and the rest of the world.

I open my heart by opening up to others: I value all interactions with other people, and I am eager to spend time building and deepening relationships, regardless of any difficulties I may encounter.

I will allow myself the experience of joy, love and happiness, and accept elements of struggle and pain that result from missed opportunities to understand others.

Bring your lover into your heart

In this exercise, you visualize an image of your partner sitting in your own heart. By bringing your mate into your heart, you activate your heart chakra. This is the most important energy centre to nourish when learning Tantric practices, because it helps unite your heart and love with your sexuality. You can practise this exercise daily to deepen your capacity for loving connection.

- Lie comfortably in the corpse pose with your arms and legs straight and relaxed, and your palms facing outwards. Alternatively, sit upright in a chair, with the soles of your feet firmly on the floor and your body relaxed. Place your hands on your knees, palms upwards.
- Become aware of your breathing, and focus on the rise and fall of your breath. Feel your body ease and your mind release.
- Now bring your attention to your partner. In your mind's eye, see an image of them as though remembering

73

a photograph. Mentally transfer this picture to the area of your heart, so that your lover sits within you. Let their image fill your heart.

- As you breathe in, send your loving breath into the centre of your heart, bathing your beloved in love. Do this for a least ten slow breaths.

Looking with love

This simple exercise is like meditation, but instead of spacing out into nothingness, you focus your attention on your mate, with an open heart. To just sit and look at each other, steadily, without blinking or looking over each other's shoulder, is challenging. The eyes are the windows to the soul, and looking creates a soul connection. Send your loving energy from your eyes into their heart.

- Sitting in easy pose with legs loosely crossed *(see page 35)*, gaze into your partner's eyes. Don't sit so close

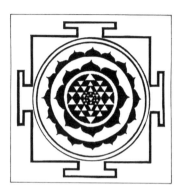

that you are unable to hold your partner's gaze comfortably for some time. Try to hold each other's gaze steadily, without letting your eyes wander over their face or around the room. This doesn't mean staring, but putting your whole being into the act of looking. As you give your attention to your lover, you also receive their gaze.

- Gaze into each other's eyes, and allow your loving feelings to emerge. It may make you feel self-conscious at first, but this is because you are still feeling separate from each other. To connect, concentrate on the love and affection that you have for your partner, rather than paying attention to your thoughts. Let your heart fill with love, and let this love overflow towards your mate.

- Just look and observe your partner, your beloved. Take in their appearance without mental comment. Still your mind, and enjoy their presence. Without speaking, look *into* your beloved, and open your heart.

Connection meditation

Meditation engenders a deeper connection with yourself and your partner. By sharing a sense of being together in the moment, cutting out external distractions, you come closer to one another. Ritual lovemaking requires that you enter a state of meditation during sex, so it's important to be able to create this mood whenever you wish. You can simply hold hands while you meditate together, or try the half-lotus. To get into this posture, sit cross-legged and bring your left foot under your right thigh. Then pick up your right foot with one hand under the right ankle and the other under the shin. While holding it, relax the leg, ensuring that it feels heavy. Then lift it and bring the heel into the angle of your left groin, with the sole of your foot facing upwards. When you are both in this position you can sit closely face to face, with each right knee resting on your partner's left knee. This lovely position circulates energy between you, creating a single unified body.

- Sit cross-legged in front of each other, or in a half-lotus. Turn the palm of your left hand upwards, to receive the palm of your partner's right hand, which is facing downwards. You can both sit in a half-lotus, dovetailing the postures with each other so that your right knee rests on your partner's left knee. You can use any of the meditations in this book: try Bringing your lover into your heart *(see page 73)* or Pelvic breathing *(see page 160)*. This is also a good posture in which to practise the tuning-in exercise below.

Tuning into your lover:
breathe together

- Lie or sit with your partner, feeling their presence and focusing on connecting sexually. Meditate on your breath, imagining that you are witnessing every in-breath and out-breath. If your mind begins to wander, keep returning your attention to your breath. The man follows the pattern of the woman's breathing.

- When you synchronize your breathing, your partner gets the message that you are really bonded. It feels as close and good as when your breathing was at one with that of your mother.

- Lie down with your back nestled into your partner's abdomen, so you mirror each other's shape like two spoons. Keep breathing together.

- For the first few minutes, focus on relaxing your body. Relax the muscles of your neck, shoulders, jaw, mouth, tongue and forehead, and around your eyes.

- Inhale through your nose, drawing in the breath steadily and gently. Breathe into your abdomen, allowing the breath to fill your abdomen slowly, by letting the chest open without your shoulders rising upwards. As you exhale gently, allow your abdomen to empty completely.

- Imagine that there are bands of energy connecting your pelvises together. Use any image that comes to mind. For example, you might imagine that both your hips are wrapped in a deep red cotton wool or that you are joined by golden gossamer threads. Alternatively, you could visualize water streaming around you or electrically charged particles dancing between you both. As you breathe in, intensify this electrical charge between you.

- Maintain a relaxed rhythm of breathing together for some minutes. Then imagine bands of energy running through your heart and into that of your lover. Visualize these bands as beams of light, coloured a warm rosy pink or a fertile, rich emerald green: these

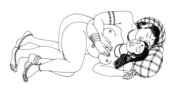

are the colours associated with the heart chakra *(see page 51)*. Feel the abundance and warmth of your joined hearts as they are held in an energy embrace. Breathe into your heart area and enjoy the feeling of contentment arising from your hearts.

- After several minutes, imagine the filaments of energy connecting your brains, like sparking wires in an electrical circuit. Send cleansing breath into both your brains with every breath. Feel your minds soften and relax. Let clear white light wash through your heads. Feel calm and peaceful together.

- Wrap your two bodies in a cocoon of brilliant light, from the tips of your toes to the tops of your heads. Relax into this rainbow light, letting your bodies absorb it and radiate light and love. Rest in the bliss.

Bonding embrace

The more close and loving you are towards your partner, the more satisfying your lovemaking. Make sure that you begin every intimate adventure with a bonding hug. You may want to play soulful, romantic music to encourage you both to open your hearts.

- Stand or lie with your arms around each other and synchronize your breathing. Melt into your lover's embrace, and feel bathed with the warmth from your lover's heart.
- Rest in your lover's arms, sinking into a heartfelt embrace. Allow yourself to feel emotionally met by your partner. Acknowledge to yourself that this is the partner whom you have chosen to be with, and appreciate the gift of love that they have brought into your life. Accept and cherish this gift.
- Appreciate the way in which your partner seems tuned into your body, and enjoy the gentle sensuality of their skin contact. Notice how their breathing mirrors yours. Sense the love pouring out towards you, and bask in its abundance.
- Relax in your lover's arms. Allow yourself the joy of feeling deeply loved. Your needs are met, so you

don't need to be needy. Let your hunger for love be satisfied.

The caressing breath

Your breath is the breath of life. Eastern cultures see the breath as the carrier of the spirit. Mingling breath is profoundly intimate.

In this exercise, you use your breath as an erotic tool, like your fingers and tongue. You use your breath to stimulate your lover's energy-body, increasing erotic sensitivity. With each exhalation, you blow softly over your lover's skin. Keep your breath deep and tender, hovering with your lips just an inch or so above the flesh.

• Begin by blowing from the base of the spine, between the buttocks, up to the base of the head. Blow from your lover's buttocks down their outstretched legs. Breathe out along the energy channels running from the heart down to the navel, and from the navel down to the genitals.

- Breathe in the fire energy around the genitals, inhaling your lover's sexual heat. Let it fill your being, nourishing you, then blow this hot energy back over their body, so your exhalation caresses the belly, top of the breasts, throat, lips and finally the forehead.

- Now that you have enlivened the principal energy conduits that link sex, the heart and the psyche, explore blowing on different parts of your lover's body. Play with your breath over their fingertips, earlobes, nape of the neck and insides of the knees.

Energy massage

The secret of Tantric massage is to energize the body while your lover is in a state of surrendered relaxation.

- Light a candle, and put on some soft background music, if music helps you to maintain a meditative state of awareness. Wash your hands before starting the massage. Then sit in silence for a few moments, centring yourself. Your partner lies down comfortably on their back, in a warm room.

- Hold your hands with palms outstretched about an inch over your lover's body. Start with small circular movements over the base of the spine and run your hands above their spine, in long, upward sweeps as you start to move the energy upwards.

- Use circular movements again in the area of the heart, between their shoulder blades. Let your hands hover above the occiput – these are the bones at the base of the head, where it sits on the neck vertebra. Focus on releasing the tension at this point while your partner imagines dark, polluted air being exhaled, releasing negative energy.

- Next, make contact with your lover's body by laying your hand on their sacrum and over their heart. After a few moments, run your palms over the skin, pausing at the navel, heart, throat and third eye, between the eyebrows.

- The next step is to press deeper into the flesh. Start at

the base of the spine and work up the back, spending some time releasing tension in the shoulders. Apply firm pressure as you both breathe in and hold it, allowing your partner to release any muscular tension, until they become still under your hands. Breathe slowly and deeply together, relaxing into this sense of stillness. Gently release the pressure, so that your partner remains relaxed.

- Once their body is relaxed, stimulate it with a fast plucking action, awakening energy in the body. Be light and playful.

- Once their body feels tingly and energized, refine their sensory sensitivity with a slow, light touch. Barely brush the skin with your fingertips. The slower you move your hands, the better this will feel.

- Next, make your massage touch even finer by using a feather. Run a feather across the skin so lightly that the very tip of the feather barely bends.

- Now eroticize the stimulation even more, while keeping it subtle. Use your hair or a silk scarf to trail across the flesh. Blow on your lover with your breath.

Appreciating your partner

Love is being loving, demonstrating your love. Love is created through loving acts. If you behave lovingly, it will bring out the best in your partner and love will grow again. The more openly you love, the more likely that loving energy will come back to you in some form. Try to give freely to your partner, without expecting reciprocation.

To foster emotional support and sustain a commitment to exploring sexual pleasure, you need to express your appreciation of each other. Make sure that your partner knows how much you value them. Stroke your partner's hair, look at them lovingly and smile: a glorious smile is linked to feelings of contentment and inner joy. Just as joy arises spontaneously, so a smile plays on your lips whenever loving thoughts about your mate warm your heart. A smile conveys your joyful mood.

The premise of a Tantric relationship is that you come together in mutual respect, freedom and honesty, and you set out to give each other pleasure. You can create an atmosphere of sacred space with your partner, in which your own body becomes a temple for worship *(see Step 3, page 101)*. Exploring your energy-body together provides an opportunity to expand hitherto neglected areas of eroticism. Even after decades of lovemaking, so many people have not developed their full sexual potential. Make a vow to make up for lost time – you can try a new exercise every night.

Once you develop your awareness, an exciting and novel area to explore is working with the subtle energy in your own body. There is tremendous potential in mixing and blending energy-bodies together with your partner, creating joy and bliss.

Touching each other's hearts

In this meditation, activate love in your heart centre in order to develop a deeper connection with your partner. By sending waves of loving energy back and forth you expand your heart energy and merge it with that of your

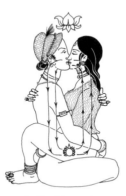

partner, making a field of love that envelopes you. This creates a bridge between your heart and sexuality, encouraging sex to be more loving.

- Choose slow, gentle, romantic music as a background aid to influence the mood.
- Close your eyes with your hands on your heart. Breathe in together while you both imagine drawing your breath through your nose and airways, down into your heart. Pause at the end of the in-breath,

focusing on your breath filling your heart. Release your breath, and slowly exhale.

- Then open your eyes, gazing at each other while continuing to breathe in harmony. Allow your loving feelings to shine from your eyes and through your breath.

- Each of you places your right hand over your partner's heart. As you exhale, imagine sending love energy from your heart down your arm and into your partner's heart. With your in-breath, imagine drawing their heart energy into your heart.

- Now breathe in as your partner breathes out. As you breathe out, they then breathe in. Through sending and receiving breath, heart energy literally circulates between you. Allow loving energy to flow out of your own body and into that of your beloved, both sharing your hearts.

Using images in lovemaking

In Tantra, mental images affirm the power of your thoughts. You can use the positive power of fantasy to create the reality you want. However, fantasies should build on what you already share. Tantra is about getting more out of what you have by going deeper into your experience. If you indulge in fantasies that take you away from your partner, your level of intimacy can only deteriorate. Imagining that you are having sex with someone else puts you in an altogether separate realm from your partner. Tantra is about remaking the universe together as a blissful experience of love.

Creative visualization means using imagery for a creative result in your lovemaking. Develop your ability to focus on mental images during sex, so that you can redefine your sexual experience, shaping and expanding it the way you want it. If you want more sexual pleasure or a whole-body orgasm *(see page 283)*, you can imagine that this is what you're having. What is in your mind partly determines how your body responds. Positive images will encourage your body to respond positively.

If you imagine the movement of energy around your body during lovemaking, then the energy will flow more easily around your body. You will feel more alive and dynamic, connecting energetically with your partner.

Fantasize about your lover

In this exercise, you use the power of your own mind to create images that enhance your joy and pleasure. Remember to maintain an awareness of your breathing as you visualize, as your breath gives power to your images.

- Close your eyes and relax your breathing. As you lie comfortably with your eyes closed, play out a scenario of lovemaking in your mind. Imagine yourself making love to your partner just as you wish. See yourself in your fantasy scenario as a sensual, erotic being. Really feel the sensations of aliveness, pleasure and desire.

- Imagine that you have all the time that you need. Your lover is taking time to pleasure you, touching you just where you want and in exactly the ways that turn you on.

- Abandon yourself to your pleasure, and see yourself in your mind's eye as sexy and satisfied.

This is an exercise that you can share with your partner, later. Try taking the opportunity to make your fantasy a reality.

Heart-to-sex breathing

Breathing and visualization exercises are designed to draw energy upwards through your body to help develop a more sensitive, subtle, evolved sexuality. The principle behind this is that your breath climbs through three chakras, or vital energy centres: the sexual centre, the heart, and the brow *(see page 51)*. By visualizing the upward movement of energy in your body, you awaken and connect these three chakras, linking your sex with your heart and spirit. You open your body to the potent energy fuelled by your erotic drive.

In this exercise, you hold a vision of love in your mind's eye and swing your energy between your hearts and genitals.

- Sit on your partner's lap or in half lotus, imagining your breath starting in your pelvis and coming up into your third eye, the area traditionally associated with inner vision. Imagine your breath rising up to this area between your eyebrows, as you visualize warm heart energy pouring into you with every in-breath. Hold a vision of love in your mind's eye, which helps you to be receptive to the energy of love. This might be a flower, a Valentine-style heart, your engagement ring, or simply a lock of hair or a tender smile. Hold this image in your mind if it helps to evoke love for your partner.

- Shift the focus of your breath back down from your heart, into your pelvis and out through your partner's genitals and into their heart. Imagine that you are swinging your breath between your two foreheads, passing through your genitals every time.

- Concentrate on creating an easy rhythm as you swing your breath back and forth between you. You can still get an erotic high from the process by letting your imagination do the work. As you breathe, let life energy stream through you. Feel the intense exhilaration of this exchange of energy with your loved one.

Variation

Once you're familiar with this combination of visualization and breathing, you'll be able to swing your heart energy between you while having intercourse: the woman sits on the man's lap with his penis inside, and you both imagine your breath dropping from your heart areas through your joined genitals and into your lover's heart, and back again.

Offering the lotus

In this ritual, you power your sexual centre by breathing in and out of your genitals, then drawing that energy into your heart to activate your love. Finally, you offer your love to your partner in a simple hand gesture. You trace the path of your breath over your body, as if offering a lotus flower as a symbol of your love.

- Stand facing each other, and gaze into each other's eyes. Let loving feelings flower as you connect with your partner.
- Inhale together, while you imagine the breath entering through your genitals. Visualize that you are breathing in through your vagina (for men, your perineum, between the anus and scrotum) and pulling the breath up through the centre of your body, coming to rest in the area of your heart by the end of each inhalation.
- Pause at the end of the in-breath, letting your sexually charged breath fill your heart. Release your breath,

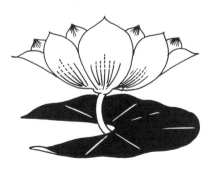

exhaling down through the centre of your body towards the tailbone and out through your genitals.

- As you continue breathing in this way for several minutes, focus on letting sexual energy build in your pelvis. With each inhalation, draw this erotic energy up to your heart with each breath. Remain in eye contact with your partner, sharing your joint desire to unite your sexuality and spirituality.

- Use your right hand to trace the progress of the energy rising from your sex into your heart. Complete the gesture by moving your hand as if you were offering a beautiful lotus flower to your partner.

- As your breath falls again, your hand can follow its pathway down the front of your body and back to your sex. This can be helpful to you both in coordinating your breathing, as you can see the path of the breath by watching the movements and rhythm of the hand rising and falling.

Special meditations and affirmations for love

Love is your essence. You're not a teacher, banker, journalist, mother or student. You're a beating heart in a living body that needs to love and be loved.

Your challenge in life is to keep your heart open in all the situations you find yourself in. Make it the top priority in your life. Love is too important to squeeze out of your life because of the pressure of work commitments. Nurture love, because you can't survive without it.

The rosebud meditation

The aim of this meditation is to feel love in your heart, and to let it spread throughout your whole being.

- With each in-breath, feel your heart opening like a rosebud. With each out-breath, allow the beauty of that open rose to permeate your body. Allow its soft scent to sweeten your soul.

- After several minutes, bring your partner to mind. If they are sitting in front of you, open your eyes slowly and gaze at them with the same feelings of loving kindness you have evoked towards yourself.

- With each in-breath, feel your heart opening. With each out-breath, send out your love to them. Feel the loving connection created between you and your breaths, and as you breathe out send out the intention that their heart flowers. Think, 'May your heart open with love.'

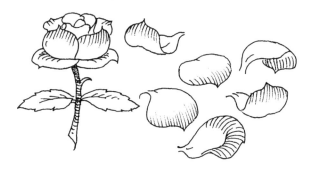

The philosophy of Tantra involves disengaging from our culture's preoccupation with romance. Lust burns itself out after a few months or years, leaving many couples washed up on an emotional desert island. You don't need to feel the heady mix of desire and fantasy associated with the early days of sexual intensity to open yourself to love and passion again. The secret is to open your own heart, rather than try to get more love from your partner.

You open to love by realizing that love is already there. You recognize the abundance of love: you don't need to feel anxious that it is a scarce resource. The nature of the universe is love, and love is always available to you.

Open to love.

Love is

In Tantra, the focus is on giving rather than on what you can get; in giving you let positive feelings flow through you, nurturing your altruistic ability to care for and love others. The more you behave in a positive way, the more those qualities will become tangible in your relationship. It's important to manifest them rather than just declare your good intentions.

- Do something loving for your partner every single day that you are together (and even when you're apart).
- Love is behaving in a way that allows your love to shine through. Acknowledge the deeper connections that remain, despite distance, disputes or temporary irritations.
- Love cannot be assumed; it must be constantly re-created in the present. Love involves constantly letting go of the past, and not being attached to future outcomes.
- Love is acceptance of what is happening between you and another, here and now.
- Make it your aim to reconnect with the love in your heart, all the time.

Getting
sensuous

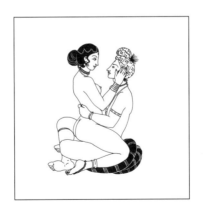

Now that you have opened your heart and connected with your partner, it is time to arouse your sexuality and refine your sensuality. We could all do with much more sensual pleasure in our lives. Daily life has become almost senseless through a sensory overload that deadens our capacity for pure pleasure.

The art of Tantra is about deepening your capacity for sensual pleasure, and acknowledging the heart connection between you. You can find more richness in your relationship by enriching it with love and giving more of yourself to it. Make your partner's needs a priority in order to make them feel deeply loved.

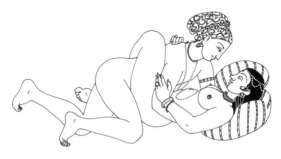

In this Step, discover the delicate, refined sensations you can treat each other to. Feel that this is an expression of your togetherness as the message of love comes through every cell in your body.

Heightening your sensual pleasure

The best sex usually occurs when you're on holiday, spending time together, feeling close and relaxed in a beautiful environment. On holiday, you are more in touch with your body: you have exercised well, and you feel physically more alive. Yet you can re-create these sensations every day with your lover. If you think about it, what you experience in life is always intense, never banal. By welcoming your experiences and surrendering to their intensity, you can heighten your sensual pleasure and learn how to arouse your lover's sensitivity in the same way.

Preparing for sensuality

Tantric exercises heighten sensitivity and awareness, and help to open your body and mind to love and excitement. Prepare whatever you need for the exercise beforehand so that your partner can just relax and concentrate on what is happening in the present moment, without thoughts or expectations. Most exercises are designed to be done by one of you first, before swapping roles.

Dance with moving awareness

Dance is a way to enjoy being in your body, appreciating the sensual pleasure of moving with abandon. In this exercise you learn how to inhabit your body and keep your attention on your bodily sensations – even when you are dancing for your partner, or with them. Dancing is like making love: you need to be inside your own experience, but connect with your partner and enjoy their body at the same time as your own. Observe the difference between focusing your attention within yourself – on your sexual centre – and outside yourself, on your partner.

- Choose a piece of music without distracting lyrics. Ideally, the music should start gently and become livelier as it progresses.
- Begin to move in a way that loosens your body and hips. Stretch your hips from side to side and gently trace shapes with your spine. Rotate your shoulders and arch your neck, stretching and relaxing the muscles.
- Begin to undulate your spine. Circle your pelvis gently and rotate your hips in a figure-of-eight movement. When you feel more relaxed and supple, start to focus your awareness inside your body. Breathe into the area of your pelvis, sensing how your body feels now it's livened up.
- Practise moving your awareness from your pelvis and then to the outside world; experiencing and then letting go; feeling excited, then detaching from the stimulating experiences you've just had.

- Start with dancing in your own style, gradually becoming slower and slower. Focus your attention within, directing your breath to your pelvis to sense the movement of energy there. Move your pelvis to help you locate the centre of your energy.

Dance for your lover's pleasure

Through dancing you can explore your unique beauty and sensuality. In this exercise, your lover can share this and enjoy it too. This treat will stimulate their visual senses.

- Enter the room wearing an outfit that makes you feel beautiful and sexy – or perhaps just a diaphanous scarf. Start by bowing to your seated partner in acknowledgement of their presence. Then forget about the fact that there is someone watching you, and abandon yourself to exploring the music. Using a long sequence of your favourite music, dance in your own unique style.

- Once you feel uninhibited and able to be adventurous, you can try exploring different moods toward your partner; for instance, dancing seductively or playfully, or in a refined or abandoned style. Try dancing with reverence for your lover, as if he were your god. If you want to invite him, he can join the dance, or take over when you want to watch him.

Snake Dance

In Tantra, your personal reservoir of energy is pictured as a snake, which sleeps coiled in your sexual centre, at the base of the spine, until charmed upward. This energy is known as *kundalini*. As you dance, you invigorate your back and pelvis, letting your energy snake up your spine. This enlivens your body, which becomes a vehicle for the expression of your passionate nature.

The Snake Dance is derived from oriental dance moves, which feel natural and easy for your body. The centre of gravity is in your hips and pelvis, and all your movements spread out from there.

- Seek out some exotic, erotic music to dance to. Arabic or Latin rhythms may inspire you, or any music that has a strong, insistent pulse.
- Start by shaking out any tension or holding around your lower back, hips, thighs and pelvis. Loosen up.
- Stand with your knees slightly bent, and trace circles with your hips as if you were dancing with a hula-hoop, but slowly. Then trace a figure-of-eight, both horizontally and vertically. Explore different angles and planes with your hip movements.
- As you dance, imagine your sexual energy awakening in your sacrum. Imagine it uncoiling like a snake climbing out of a snake charmer's basket and dancing up your spine, embracing the sexual energy of your lover. Embrace your lover as you move.
- Let your erotic, snake-like bodies dance together.

Variation: Dance as foreplay to lovemaking

One of the secrets of Tantric sex is to make love with your partner from a mood of relaxed excitement and then move into a state of heightened sensitivity. Rather than use sex to arouse your sexual energy, practise awakening your desire through dance. Once your body is singing with the pleasure of movement, you can relax into the erotic pleasures of being alive and share this joy with your partner.

Make love to music

Let the pleasure of music invite you to surrender to your senses. Think about the mood that you want to evoke; muse on the music that you find relaxing, intimate, exciting or seductive. You can choose one of the available Tantra CDs for lovemaking, or compile your own tape or CD. Think about your patterns of arousal, excitement and times spent connecting during lovemaking, and choose your lovemaking music together.

When first exploring Tantra it is helpful to play spacious, slow and romantic music that facilitates timeless emotional bonding rather than fast, driving music that suggests fucking. Lyrics that emphasize love, connection and a celebration of aliveness might appeal, but beware distracting pop tunes that may bring up memories and moods associated with past experiences and relationships – and may not help you focus on what you're doing in the present moment.

Music needs to encourage the build-up of emotional and sexual energy between the two of you right now, rather than inviting comparisons with past lovers. You want it to help you keep distraction at bay and help you fully focus on the connection with your lover. Rhythms that synchronize with your heartbeat or breathing patterns will help harmonize you. Hypnotically repetitive New Age music might be very calming if you tend to have a busy mind that intrudes into your lovemaking. A powerful base beat stimulates your erotic drive for sexual pleasure.

It's ideal if you can find music or create a tape that starts gently with plenty of time for bonding and sensual exploration, becoming more dynamic as you make love and then slowing into a more contemplative mood during the afterglow.

Bedroom bliss

In this ritual you create a sanctuary of bliss that inspires lovemaking. Aim to make your environment evoke a dreamy, playful mood. You may wish to re-create the flavour of your last holiday together, playing music that reminds you of your time away and placing items around the room that you bought there. Whatever theme you choose, convert your bedroom into a beautiful temple of love.

- Cleanse your space. Tidy away clutter, disconnect the telephone and cover up any work-related objects such as computers or files. Clean free surfaces, and re-make your bed with fresh, inviting linen. As you work, leave the windows open and encourage all distractions, stress and worry to float away. The more you clean and tidy, the calmer your psychic and physical space becomes.

- Ornament the room with flowers and sculpted objects that feel nice to touch – stones, shells, feathers.
- Choose calm, relaxing music to create a smooth ambience. Plan several tracks ahead, so you won't need to pay attention to anything else but your lover.
- Lighting should be subtle and indirect. Use table lamps, or set up candles in a safe place where they won't easily be disturbed.
- Scent the room by burning incense or essential oils. Alternatively, add a few drops of essential oil to an atomizer of warm water and spray a fine mist round the room.
- Robe yourself and your lover in soft, sensual fabrics; wear a silky dressing gown, kimono or sarong.

Loving your lover's body

Following a Tantric path to sensual pleasure means becoming more attentive to your senses and to those of your partner. Physically caring for your lover arouses their sensitivity, creating more intimacy in your relationship. If you have not been sufficiently appreciative of your lover's body in the past, you may need to pay positive attention to them now in order to heal any lingering feelings of low self-esteem.

- Light a candle so that you are both bathed in warm, flattering light.
- Slowly undress your partner, gently and with love. Gaze upon them appreciatively as you strip away their clothing. Use words and gestures that honour their naked body in the way you now honour your own. Show them that you love them as you love yourself, through the temple of your body. The mood of this ritual is to honour sexuality as a sacred expression of your love.

113

Essential oils for love

In your sacred space, choose essential oils that soothe the nervous system and enhance erotic feelings. Try ylang-ylang, lavender or any others whose aroma appeals to you both.

Ylang-ylang is sweet and sensuous

Lavender is relaxing and cleansing

Sandalwood and frankincense create a meditative atmosphere

Geranium is relaxing and uplifting

Rose enhances love and sensuousness

Bergamot is refreshing

Jasmine creates a richly sumptuous atmosphere.

Erotic touch

This is not a prelude to lovemaking, but it fulfils the desire for sensual touch independent of sexual contact. Use touch to intrigue your lover and tantalize the sensory receptors in their skin. You'll need some delicate feathers to trail across your lover's body.

• Make sure that the room is warm and set it up with soft, sensual music playing. Ask your partner to lie down naked, either on their back or on their front.

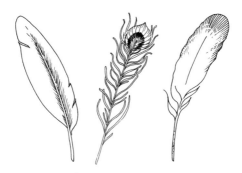

- Stroke their body gently with a feather, starting around the shoulders and throat, then moving gradually and sensuously down the body to the feet, and finishing with the head. Then use your fingertips, and lastly your breath, blowing about an inch away from the body. If you keep the contact with the feather as continuous as possible, your partner can relax into the delicate sensation.

- Keep your touch very light and as slow as possible. Treat your partner's body as a whole rather than focusing on erogenous zones. Breathe over the sacrum bone. Direct your breath along the curve of their spine, tracing the line from the tailbone, tucked between tight buttocks, up to the small of the back.

- When receiving your lover's breath, concentrate on receiving its heat. Warm your body with it. Allow your muscles to melt as if their breath were igniting your fire.

Tantalize your lover

This exercise is a Tantric interpretation of the tasting game, but your lover is enchanted and tantalized by sensational touch, taste and the tone of your voice. When blindfolded, there are no distractions to interfere with the immediacy of their experience. You carefully stimulate each sense in turn, and your lover savours each sensory impression with a sensual pleasure enhanced by being blindfolded. Spend an hour or so on this exercise, leaving a minute or two between each stimulus.

• Create your temple of love *(see Bedroom bliss, page 111)*, decorating your room with beautiful items that have meaning for you both. Then collect together all the ingredients you will need: a tray of morsels for taste, feathers or fur for touch, a bell or singing bowl for sound, essential oils to stimulate the sense of smell. Light the candles and incense, and place the food tray in the centre of the room in an aesthetic arrangement together with all the other objects you will use.

Blindfold your partner and gently lead them into the room. They have nothing to do but breathe, relax and enjoy the experiences you offer them – preferably without talking.

- *Harmonics:* Rather than create a cacophony of sound, begin with one note or vibration. Choose a short excerpt from an atmospheric CD, or gently clap a simple rhythm. If you have any musical instruments such as drums, bells, flutes or maracas you can use these. Make this first sound as continuous and resonant as possible. For example, make a singing bowl sing by striking it and running the mallet around the rim, or ring a bell softly – you can move around your partner as you do this.

- *Aroma:* Take a bottle of unstoppered essential oil and hold it under your partner's nose without contacting the skin. Allow them to inhale for a few seconds, then wait a minute before offering the next smell. Peppermint or eucalyptus essence is good to start with, followed by sweeter and more mysterious essences such as ylang-ylang, jasmine and gardenia.

- *Touch:* Brush your lover's skin with fur or fabric. You can use the corner of a rug, a tasselled cushion, a fur collar. Then play their skin with feather, silk, velvet or satin. Move it slowly and delicately across the cheeks, neck and arms – or wrists and ankles.

- *Taste:* Tempt your lover with an offering of exotic fruit, such as lychees, mango, star fruit, passion fruit or kiwi fruit. Feed them by hand, little by little. Offer a sip from a glass of sparkling elderflower wine or cordial. You can dip your finger into a liqueur and caress your partner's lips with it. Tease and tantalize – dip a little kiwi fruit into liqueur, then press it to your partner's lips, letting the taste linger before you introduce it to their tongue.

- *Sight:* To finish, silently remove your partner's blindfold. Gaze at each other for a few minutes, and at the tableau of objects and ingredients that you have used to create your sensory journey. You might like to embrace, feeling your lover's body melt into yours.

119

Sensational sex

The secret of Tantric sex is to make an energetic connection with your lover, rather than trying to fulfil emotional or physical needs. Because emotions are so transitory – and often get in the way of a heart connection – concentrate instead on intensifying your sensory perceptions. You can have sensational sex by going deeper inside your body and identifying with the delectable sensations it provides. Learn to sink into the feelings, sensations and surges of energy that arise in your body during lovemaking. Let love awaken and activate your energy-body.

If you feel your mind wandering during sex, bring it back to what you are doing and focus on the sensations in your body. Bring your attention back to the quality of emotional connection between you, sensing the nature of your pleasure, arousal and love: are these feelings delicate, or consuming?

Sensuous love postures

Be spontaneous and adventurous in your lovemaking. Surprise your lover by suggesting a sexual prelude before going out, or using a sitting-up posture to make love rather than lying down. If you want to make love upright, you can move into the yab-yom position (named after the Tibetan statues of gods and goddesses wrapped in a sexual embrace) where the woman sits on her partner's lap with her legs wrapped around him. In this position, the man can't thrust as much (unless his partner leans back and rests on her hands) so it is perfect for slow, sensual lovemaking, breathing together and visualization. It's ideal for circling your breath through your joined lips *(see page 309)* and for having a whole-body orgasm *(see page 283)*.

Making love when you're both upright means that you are equally active sexually. When you are wrapped around each other, your sexual union symbolizes the union of bliss and compassion, technique and soulfulness. When the two aspects are merged within, you

move together into the non-dual, formless realm of bliss
– see Step 7 for more on this blissful state.

Voice your desire during lovemaking

Traditionally, Tantra uses a lot of chants, humming and
devotional singing to harness the power of your mind to
move energy through your body and open your sexual
response. We explored one of these exercises, Relax and
chant, in Step 1 *(see page 9)*.

Your voice is therefore one of the keys to enhanced
sexual pleasure. It is hard to abandon yourself in lovemaking if your lips are tightly sealed. Being vocal enhances the
connection between you and your partner; we know this
through the simple fact that we feel closer to friends when
we talk and share our experiences. Verbalizing bodily
sensations as they arise also accentuates pleasure. Try not
to think too much, as thinking tends to distance you from
the directness of your experience. Remain identified with
your feelings, rather than analysing them.

- Experiment with the difference between lying with your mouth closed and letting your head loll back in a gesture of abandon, extending your throat and opening your mouth. Let sound come out without censoring it. If you find this difficult at first, start by magnifying the sound and gesture that you want to make. Overacting can start you off, and help you lose your inhibitions. This is an especially good idea when your genitals are being stimulated.

- Your sounds of pleasure give your partner feedback about what delights you. It also keeps their attention engaged so that they don't wander off into their own thoughts. Best of all, it's a massive form of arousal for the listener. When you can hear how much pleasure you are giving your partner you feel good about yourself, which arouses your own sexuality.

- Voicing your pleasure through sighs, moans, groans and yelling enhances your excitement. You can even turn yourself on just through making noises as if you were highly aroused. Your body will follow the cues given by your verbal anticipation.

Using the five senses during lovemaking

Senses are the link between your subtle, pre-verbal experience and the outer world of connecting and relating.

To fully appreciate your lover, become absorbed in their sensational body.

1 During lovemaking, taste your lover's sexual juices. Get in the mood where you find them irresistibly yummy.
2 Inhale the whole scent of your lover into your being, as if incorporating them through your nose. If you enjoy the smell of their sweat, sexual fluids or perfume, let that satiate your sense of smell.
3 Arouse your lover with different qualities of touch. Enjoy the texture of satin sheets, feathers *(see page 115)* or any interesting tactile objects that you can use to sensitize your lover. The simple sensation of soft touch on the skin can be extremely powerful.
4 Arouse your partner's sense of hearing with seductive comments about what you're doing and how you

intend to titivate them, or how they make you feel and how you feel about them.

5 To arouse their sense of vision, lead your lover through a guided fantasy – let your imagination roam. Invent scenarios that you enjoy as well as those that turn them on, so that you both share this fantastical erotic journey.

Open up to erotic pleasure during lovemaking

People with good sex lives feel that they are entitled to sexual satisfaction. They assume that enjoying sex is natural, not an optional extra in a relationship. To realize your capacity for erotic pleasure, you need to feel confident about receiving pleasure. Remember that pleasure is your birthright: you deserve it.

In this exercise you take turns receiving. Your partner agrees to do whatever you desire. As you accept sensory stimulation, concentrate on incorporating the pleasure into your being. Let the experience nurture you. However, make sure that you don't turn this wonderful opportunity into a power-trip. It is an occasion to unreservedly go for what you want, because you know that your partner has the option of saying no if they don't fancy doing something specific. But the agreement is that they will try to go along with whatever you wish to support you in exploring the scope of your erotic desires. Feel grateful when your lover complies with your requests, and enjoy the experience of having your sexual preferences recognized and attended to.

- Ask directly and simply for what you want without hesitation or manipulation.
- As you ask your lover to do pleasurable things for you and to you, enjoy the feeling of being enabled to express your desires. State your wishes without requiring that your partner complies with them.
- Although you are directing your own lovemaking session, enter a receptive mode. Relax and open yourself to sensual pleasure from your lover. As your

partner touches you, feel how your body is enlivened and stimulated by their full attention. Focus on the energy released within you under your lover's touch. Let the energy flow through your body, and let go of any expectations. Without expectation there can be no frustration, disappointment or bitterness about not having your needs met.

- Remind yourself that you are worthy of receiving. Acknowledge to yourself that your sensual needs are being met, and notice how much pleasure this brings you. Allow yourself to enjoy receiving; feel nourished by your partner's giving.

- Focus on your endless capacity for enjoyment, while you are touched and pleasured. Sink into your pleasure.

Pleasuring your partner

Pleasure your partner in the ways that he or she enjoys, while asking for feedback, guidance and affirmation that what you are doing is appropriate. In order to serve your partner in a way that nourishes them, you need to tune into their needs, immersing yourself in what you are doing for, and with, them. If you feel your mind wandering, look at their face (and into their eyes, if they are open), imparting love through your gaze.

While touching your partner, keep the channels of communication open. Ask for their guidance; ask what they want; ask how it feels. Encourage them to describe their inner state. Appreciate this high level of communication.

- Start by stroking and stimulating your lover's whole body. Rather than going straight for the genitals, touch, kiss and caress their flesh, enjoying the texture, pressure and movement of sexual energy as you arouse them.
- You can explore any of the tips in this book, including massage, erotic touch, awakening the senses, sensory massage, genital massage, g-spot stimulation and oral sex.

Creative lovemaking

Most of us learn how to make love from our earliest sexual experiences, before we had the confidence to fully explore our own unique sexual preferences. Some of us carry on making love in the same way, without exploring all the possibilities available in the language of lovemaking. In order to expand your sexual repertoire,

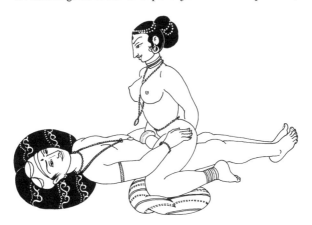

take nothing for granted – regardless of how many times you have made love together – and be adventurous about trying out anything that appeals to you both.

Creativity is about finding your own personal voice – it doesn't have to be different or original. It's a good idea to explore a whole range of sensual and sexual feelings

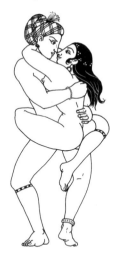

to find out what feels most comfortable to you. You don't need to strive but instead adopt an attitude of playful openness. Through lovemaking you can mutually discover new aspects of yourselves that you had excluded from your sexual identities, bringing you self-acceptance and peace.

Explore the fantasies that you find erotically seductive. Discuss the fantasies that you cherish, to see whether you are both happy exploring them together. Think about what characters or dress styles intrigue and appeal. You might be attracted to the medieval era of courtly love, the carnival play with masked disguise used in Venice, or Middle Eastern attitudes towards the voracity of women's sexual appetites. You might want to discuss a scenario with your partner in order to come up with ideas and details together.

Make love for the first time

Do you recall the first time you had sex? The anticipation. The excitement and intensity. And, of course, the uncertainty, that feeling of not knowing what to do or what to expect. In first-time sex, you explore someone else's body and genitals without preconceptions.

Remember seeing the signs of sexual arousal: the wetness and engorgement, the mixture of fear, breathlessness, heat, tentativeness. In this exercise you recapture the sense of novelty without the anxiety that is often associated with making love for the first time.

- Touch your partner tentatively, not as if you already know where to touch, but in an exploratory manner, as if you want to find out what will open your partner to you sexually and give them pleasure.
- Discover what makes your lover's body move toward you (wanting more) or away (wanting less of the same stimulation). Experiment with different styles of touch; vary the pressure and pace. Whereas the first time you had sex you probably didn't talk about what you were doing, often literally groping in the dark, you now have the benefit of communication skills acquired over the course of your relationship. Ask what your lover is feeling in response to your touch.

Now you're making love without a script; it's not an automated repeat of previous performances with little variation. After all, your mood is different each time you come together, just as your love is re-created afresh each and every moment together.

STEP FOUR

Sexual power: explore your desire

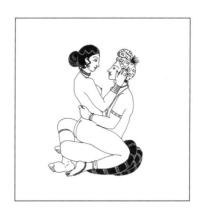

Now that you have nourished your sensual self, discover your sexual self. Your sexuality encompasses a whole range of qualities, such as eroticism, playfulness, excitement, tenderness and ardour. When you express your sexual energy, you step into your personal power.

The drive for sexual expression produces desire. In Tantric sex, you harness your sexual desire to your heart energy, imbuing your lust with love. You can create a conscious link between these two poles of your sexuality by moving energy from your sexual centre into your heart during lovemaking. This is a secret Tantric practice that makes sex explosively powerful.

You can also use your emotional connection with your partner to awaken your sexual self. If you move your relationship to centre stage in your life and make sex the pivot of your relationship, you can use the potent combination of love and sex to make bliss your daily reality.

The suggestions in this Step are to be approached in a spirit of fun. Learn to lighten up, and add sweetness to your relationship. Put more heart into it. Have a laugh about what you are trying out, recapturing an innocent sense of fun, wonder and joy. Laughter is bonding, because it is a recognition that you are together in this sexual exploration. However you communicate, you need to be open and honest about your desires. Give each other feedback about what works for you: say what you enjoyed about the things you experimented with. In taking responsibility for discussing your personal experience with your partner, you create an atmosphere of love and trust.

Firing your passion

Tantric techniques are all about igniting your fire energy – powering your energy-body with the fire of your sexual passion, and then transforming your two energy-bodies into a single body of bliss. You can open your heart by learning to channel the force of your sexual passion, holding its heat in your heart until emotionally you burst into ardent flames. The flames from this fire will burn through all the obstacles in your relationship to make it stronger and more vital.

What is desire?

Desire is an expression of your libido, your zest for life. It is a primal means of engaging with the world around you. Most spiritual traditions try to sublimate desire because of the tendency to get overattached to the object of your desire. This is considered to be the fundamental cause of suffering. Tantra encourages you to really live out your desire without being attached to its form or goal. In other words, you can truly enjoy the experience of desiring, rather than treating desire as a goal. Specific goals always elude us, while that of desiring can enrich our lives and make our relationship sparkle with promise. Desire gives your interaction spice and flavour.

Desire is ...

I can allow myself to experience all my emotions.

I accept my longing.

I reclaim my sexuality.

I resolve guilt-demons.

Guilt is a pleasure-killer. It arises out of low self-esteem, which can damage sexuality. Guilt can manifest itself as dissociation between sex and love, or a desperate searching for love through compulsive sex. The exercises in this book can help heal hurt or guilt from the past that gets in the way of expressing your desire *(see also Step 5, page 175)*.

A meditation on desire

- Imagine that your body is made of desire. Visualize desire as a warm or hot colour – molten gold, or the sparks of a bonfire irradiating your body. Let the fire blaze and its heat emanate. Feel full of warmth and joy.
- Let the gold pour through your whole body, permeating every pore and cell. Let molten gold stream through you and clear out all the debris of your life.
- Feel saturated with desire. Imagine your body sparkling with it.

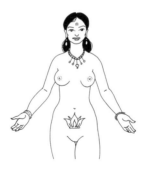

Reigniting desire

When you open your heart and join it with that of your lover, you are both entering the flame of love. Allow the fire of your passionate nature, and the intensity of your experience, to encourage you to love each other without any reservation or holding back. You can choose to create this passion with your partner, even if you feel that your relationship has lost its chemistry. By deciding to rebuild your relationship in this way, you can transform your twosome into an incandescent dance of energy. Even with the most familiar partner you can reconnect with your vital erotic impulse. You do this by first working on yourself, by reactivating your loving and passionate nature.

If you find that you can barely summon love for your partner, turn this around by actively deciding to reclaim love. Remember that love is continually created through loving acts. If you behave lovingly, it will bring out the best in your partner and love will grow once again. The more openly you love, the more likely that loving energy will come back to you from your partner. Try to give to them freely without expecting that they reciprocate. This creates a more inviting atmosphere between you.

The premise of a Tantric relationship is that you come together in mutual respect, freedom and honesty. Giving each other pleasure is high on your agenda. Reaffirm this commitment to provide pleasurable opportunities every day, in sexual and other ways. Agree to extend your sexual repertoire – explore the far reaches of your sexual capacities and find your sexual fulfillment with each other.

If your lovemaking has become predictable

If you feel that your sexuality is dormant or that you've been getting into a predictable lovemaking routine, you may want to schedule plenty of time to explore different aspects of both your sexualities. You need time to be free to experiment. You may want to give in to lust or explore your fantasies through imaginative play, or learn to improve your sexual repertoire and deepen your soul connection. Whatever it is you want to explore, make sex a priority – schedule an hour of pleasure every night. What could be more enjoyable than spending time making love?

Exploring boundaries

The following three exercises deal with setting up helpful sexual boundaries by making agreements to meet each other's need for sex, and committing to stopping sex whenever it doesn't feel right for you. You can also show your lover how to stimulate you through pleasuring yourself in front of them. Through sharing and caring for each other in this way, you foster qualities of sensitivity, consideration, nurturing and love, helping you to get the best out of your sexual relationship.

Meeting each other's needs for sex

Make an agreement that in principle you will always be responsive to each other's needs. Agree not to refuse each other sex. This is a good strategy to avoid power games in which sex is bartered or withheld. It also means that you can feel more confident about approaching your partner, knowing that you are unlikely to be rebuffed. Unless your sexual needs are way out of synch and only one of you wants to have sex all the time, agree to make love with your partner whenever there is an erotic charge between you.

If your levels of desire are very different, it's a good idea to find new ways to connect through meditation, breathing and visualization before you reintroduce intercourse *(see pages 15, 35)*. All these techniques are perfect whenever you feel disconnected for some reason. Making a sex agreement doesn't imply that you agree to make love in ways you're not happy with. What it does mean is making a commitment to keep your sexual connection alive and thriving, and working on improving it if it is not satisfying for either of you. Use your agreement as a way to welcome even more erotic pleasure into your lives.

Show your partner what excites you

The best way to ensure your sexual satisfaction is to learn how to get your sexual needs met. If you don't know what these are, you need to explore them on your own. Once you have found out what turns you on, you can demonstrate it to your partner so they can include some of your preferred techniques in their repertoire of pleasuring skills. This intimate exercise is also good for deepening trust.

- If you have the nerve, invite your partner to witness a whole session of self-pleasuring. Self-pleasure your pearl (clitoris) or penis for half an hour or so, so that they observe how you touch yourself and learn what you enjoy.
- Let your partner take over, while you tell him or her what feels good and how to touch you. Or they can invent strokes and rhythms to find new approaches.

Agreeing to stop

Make an agreement with your partner that you immediately stop what you're doing whenever one person
feels upset during sex – whenever they feel detached,
numb, upset, angry or bored. This doesn't mean that
you should pull away physically or withdraw your
penis. Just bond, with your arms wrapped around one
other, letting your partner share these emotions with
the reassurance that they won't lose your love by
expressing them. Your partner needs to feel that their
distress is acknowledged and dealt with, rather than
ignored. Don't just carry on as if you are not feeling
upset or disengaged. Suppressing your difficulties will
damage the emotional and energetic connections
between you both, and lead to further wounding or
cutting off.

If you can't deal with the feelings and need to stop
intimate contact, you need to tell your partner exactly
how you would like them to support you. Think about
what would help you process these feelings and

hopefully clear them, so that you can get back to love-making in a gentle, sensitive and connected way.

Saying 'yes' and 'no' during lovemaking

You have to know that you are able to say no to anything that you don't want sexually in order to be able to say 'yes' without reservation. Playing the 'yes'/'no' game helps you take charge of meeting your own needs for sexual pleasure. Saying 'yes' to pleasure – or 'no' – may be equally difficult for people who are not used to talking about sex. This is an exercise in clear, unambiguous communication.

During a session of intimate contact and sexual exploration, you agree that you will respond with one or two words to everything that your partner does to you. Choosing 'yes' or 'no' means that you have to state a preference – you can't remain equivocal about the way your partner touches you. Sometimes you may feel you don't know your desires well enough, so you go along with whatever your partner suggests. It's important to clearly communicate your sexual needs by saying 'yes' to what you do want and enjoy. It is equally important, if not more so, to be able to say 'no' to what you don't want. It is very difficult to be sexually open and exploratory if you feel under pressure to make love in ways that risk alienating you.

- During a session in which your partner explores different ways of pleasuring you, communicate using 'yes' or 'no'.
- Depending upon your intonation, 'yes' can mean: *I like that, I want more, keep going.* 'No' can mean: *I'm not sure, I really don't like that, stop doing what you're doing.*

Saying yes to pleasure

If it is tricky saying no, it can be even more difficult to say yes. However, it is important to be unreservedly enthusiastic about experiencing pleasure if you want to get the most out of sex. Through pleasure you affirm your bodily existence, and you cannot have too much of it. You deserve pleasure.

In this exercise, your partner gives you a massage while you concentrate on maximizing your feelings of pleasure. This helps release the tension in your body left over from armouring it against possible stress or pain. When you hold feelings in your body in this way, the tension reduces your capacity for pleasurable impressions. When you're giving pleasure, make it a practice to focus on your partner without thinking about your own sexual needs. Concentrate wholeheartedly on giving your partner pleasure rather than being distracted by your own desire.

- Your lover starts by massaging your abdomen. This relaxes and releases the abdominal muscles, softening your belly and the source of your erotic energy, and preparing your pelvis to open up on more subtle levels.
- As your partner delicately strokes you, bask in his

undivided attention. Focus on accepting pleasure into your whole being. He can blow hot breath over your skin for several minutes, and then slowly stroke you with a feather for several minutes more. Using the tips of his fingers very slowly and sensitively, he makes light contact with the surface of your skin.

- Just enjoy being touched without having to reciprocate. What's important is simply to experience the moment, with no deferral of fulfilment to the future. You don't have to do anything in return. This massage is just for you.

- Tell your partner when you want them to touch your genitals sexually, or if you would prefer them to move their hands away from your abdomen and massage the rest of your body. Tell your lover how you want to be touched, and where.

- Try saying 'Yes' out loud each time your lover touches you in a delightful way to give yourself permission to luxuriate in the sensations as they arise. If saying yes is too embarrassing, try saying a long 'Ah', releasing your breath in a relaxed way with each thrill.

Focus on the difference between
giving and taking

Learn how to give without the expectation of receiving anything in return. You can do this in small ways by presenting gifts to show your appreciation (whether flowers, cards or poems) and taking the time to care for your lover's personal needs. Be generous. Enjoy giving – be aware of what is important to your partner, and do helpful things for them. Take your own pleasure from pleasuring your partner and witnessing their enjoyment.

While it is appropriate for your partner to communicate their wishes to you rather than expecting you to know what they want, you are not responsible for meeting all their needs. Nor is it up to you to try to guess what your partner feels or wants at all times. However, it's a pleasure when they sense that you are attuned to them and enjoy giving them the gift of time and attention. The experience of giving is very different when it is a result of your choice rather than an obligation.

The structure is very simple. Agree a period of time in

which one of you asks for what you want, and describes exactly how you would like it to be. You might simply want to be nurtured or taken care of. You might want your lover to run a bath for you, cook for you or massage you while you relax. You might want your partner to make love to you while you just lie back and enjoy it. It's up to you – you say what you want.

- When you are giving, try to remain tuned in and sensitive to the needs of your partner, focusing on them one hundred per cent. It's not necessary to do anything you don't want to do. If you feel your partner is asking for something that makes you uncomfortable, just say so and offer to do something else.

- When you are receiving, as you feel your partner's touch, concentrate totally on the pleasure and allow yourself to relax into the subtle physical sensations. Let go of any resistance or withholding due to a fear of being let down or disappointed, or anxiety about the outcome of the session. Revel in the attention.

Being active and passive in sex

What is the difference in the quality of your experience between being the doer and the done-to? In this exercise, you alternate between active and passive roles during lovemaking. You can fine-tune your sexual

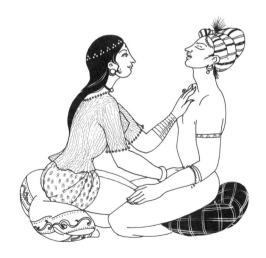

pleasure to make sure that one of you is stimulated more if your arousal levels are dropping, rather than one of you forging ahead and leaving the other behind. It is desirable to be able to pace your sexual arousal until you get to the point of choosing when to have a simultaneous orgasm. However, it's also a good opportunity to completely let go of taking responsibility for giving your partner pleasure, rather than both of you compromising because you are trying to please each other and get your own erotic pleasure at the same time.

In this practice, you take charge of your own sexual satisfaction. Men can let go of the performance imperative – making love in a woman-on-top position is a good way for the man to give up control. The woman can enjoy orchestrating her genital pleasure and the pace of intercourse.

• Try to spend at least forty minutes with one of you active while the other laps up the pleasure. Then swap over so that the passive partner stimulates the other. Over the course of a lovemaking session you will find out how long you can each give pleasure for before your erotic interest wanes, letting an easy rhythm of alternation develop.

- Keep checking on how your partner is doing, and give them your feedback.
- When you and your partner become totally tuned to one another, you will no longer think about who is doing the pleasuring; your roles disappear as you become totally immersed in your shared joy.

Communicating during sex

It's revealing for your partner when you spell out what sex feels like for you. Your partner doesn't automatically know what you feel or what you want – your desires are not necessarily the same as theirs, so you can't take anything for granted. This practice is aimed at conveying information about your subjective experience of sex – which can be a revelation. It's the ultimate in communication.

In this exercise you describe your experience during

sex so that your lover finds out how you feel during each and every stage of your lovemaking. You simply relate your feelings, sensations and emotions as they arise. You can do this together or take turns during consecutive rounds of sex.

- Describe your experience without reservation as an uninhibited stream of consciousness. In this way, you let your partner know precisely how you feel during lovemaking.
- You can take the opportunity to share information about what arouses you, and let your partner know if their attempts fail to excite you. Be sensitive to their response. Your emotional communication will open up, because of the trust involved in sharing this degree of sexual detail.
- Your partner can help by asking questions to elicit more description. It's good for your partner to have the opportunity to say how they felt listening to you. Try to accept what they say without much comment *(see also Active listening, page 200)*.

Exchanging love and energy

Sex is something that two people create together – an energetic exchange as well as physical interaction. Sex involves a complex of elements, including emotion, desire, connection, need, longing, pleasure, movement, sensation and smell. Tantric sex involves heart, breath, inner vision, body and soul. The combination of all of these aspects creates a powerful holistic experience. In order to foster qualities of openness, sensitivity and a whole-body eroticism, focus on the quality of your heart connection. Sense your lover's heart in your whole being. This opens you up to a true Tantric experience.

Understanding the energy dimension of sex further enriches your erotic life. Sex is an exchange of energies, not just body fluids. Learn to experience the subtle energies that are exchanged as you make love.

Being orgasmic

Your sexual nature is orgasmic. Orgasm is more than the pleasurable muscular contractions in your vagina and pelvis that bring a feeling of release; among other things it incorporates heat, arousal, desire, love and connection. In Tantra, orgasm plugs you into an altered state of consciousness in which you experience the world as bliss. Your birthright is bliss, just as your nature is orgasmic.

Couples often need to garner more sexual techniques in order to have regular orgasms and improve their sex life. You both need regular sexual satisfaction before you can let go of the goal of orgasm and explore non-orgasmic sexual pleasure. Women who consistently find it easy to orgasm say the following.

- That the key to regular orgasm is feeling sexy and desirable. Their attitude is that they deserve to have an orgasm.
- That their partners are willing to spend extra time

stimulating them before going on to have intercourse – at least half an hour of genital stimulation.

- They feel confident enough to guide their partner, showing them how to pleasure them most effectively.
- During oral sex, orgasmic women feel that it's good to concentrate on receiving pleasure rather than trying to give to their partner at the same time. They tell themselves that he's enjoying licking them as much as they are enjoying the attentions of his tongue.
- That they stimulate their clitoris themselves if they need extra stimulation during intercourse in order to reach a climax.

If you have difficulty reaching orgasm, the first task in exploring your sexuality is to discover how to realize your orgasmic potential. It is important to learn how to achieve orgasm through self-pleasuring, then sharing this knowledge with your partner and incorporating it into your lovemaking before going on to Tantric breathing and visualization techniques *(see Step 1, page 59, for ideas on self-stimulation)*. Tantric orgasm is really the icing on the cake; learning to expand from genital orgasm into whole-body orgasm and then how to use orgasmic streamings to enter the slipstream of your unified energy. When the energy pours out of both your bodies you feel connected with your beloved in an ocean of universal love. Now, that's ultimate bliss!

The anatomy of desire

Tantric wisdom has a great deal of insight about the physical and energy processes in lovemaking. When your heart is energized a feeling of strength, passion and aliveness arises in your being and nourishes your capacity to relate. Closing down your feelings about yourself produces apathy and depression.

Tantra sees your desire as a manifestation of your energy-body and uses the metaphor of fire to work with it. Fire needs to be started with small pieces of kindling. As it is fed, the flames grow bigger, heading straight upward and engulfing everything along the way.

Tantrics believe that once you have awakened your sexual energy, you should encourage your desire to climb up from your genitals, imbuing your heart with passion, your mind with insight and the crown of your head with bliss.

Pelvic techniques in Tantra

The following pelvic and pelvic breathing exercises are designed to awaken your erotic impulse and use it to stoke the fire. Of course, in theory you don't really need to follow exercises on what to do or how to live your life – from one perspective that's contrary to the spirit of Tantra, which recommends going with the flow rather than doing anything formulaic. These exercises are intended as a springboard for your own creative sexual energy, helping you to cultivate a different attitude towards lovemaking. Once you've become aware of where in your being your energy needs to be focused, you can respond intuitively to the mood between you. By developing awareness about working with the subtle

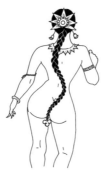

energy in your own body, you can mix and blend energy-bodies together with your partner to create something marvellous.

Pelvic breathing for sexual fire

Tantrics use this heavy-breathing meditation to awaken sexual energy, building a fiery sexual charge in your body. You can practise this alone or with your partner, as a preliminary to lovemaking.

- Sit cross-legged. Focus on your breath dropping down to your belly. Let your belly open and expand with each in-breath. Let your body release as the breath moves down.
- After a few moments, take in three or four short quick breaths through your nose then relax your breathing on the long out-breath. Try to send the quick breaths down into your belly – you may hyperventilate slightly when doing this, so replenish your oxygen supplies by alternating rapid breathing with slow, deep, belly breaths at any point. Try rounds of short, gasping breaths with a longer series of deep, belly breaths for at least ten or fifteen minutes.
- If you are sitting cross-legged before your partner, synchronize the sequence of slow, deep breathing and short gasping breaths so that you breathe together.

It can be vitalizing to dance straight after this exercise *(see Step 3, pages 104–106)*, enhancing the energy that has started to move in your body.

Pelvic floor exercises

Improving the tone of your pelvic floor muscles, or 'love muscles', can do wonders for your sex life. It makes it easier for you to orgasm and to control the build-up to orgasm. The pelvic floor muscles are the same ones that women are encouraged to exercise after giving birth! In men, squeezing the pelvic floor muscles around the base of your penis and anus may produce a rise. If you are semi-erect you can practise moving your penis up and down as you squeeze your love muscle. Strengthening these muscles also cultivates confidence in your physical flexibility and helps create an awareness of your erotic energy. When your love muscles are really strong, you can squeeze your vagina to massage your lover's penis while he is inside you. You will notice that when you squeeze your love muscles, you feel pleasurable sensations in your genitals.

At first it is best to do this exercise while lying down, so you can concentrate on the pelvic floor muscles. When you've become adept, you can practise the exercise anywhere. You need to do dozens every day for a few months in order to fully tone these muscles. The basic exercise is as follows:

- Lie on the floor with your spine aligned and your knees bent upward. The only muscular stress you feel should be along your inner thighs as they support your knees – the rest of your body should feel relaxed.
- Lengthen your spine and stretch your neck, tucking your chin in toward your chest.
- As you breathe in, squeeze your pelvic floor muscles – it can help to imagine that you are slowly pulling up your jeans zip from the base of your crotch to your midriff. Hold your breath for a moment and, as you inhale, allow your filling abdomen to push the zip down without any effort on your part – just allow the muscles to release.
- Every day, spend at least ten minutes breathing into your pelvic floor muscles as a zip that you pull up and down. Regular exercise strengthens these muscles and enhances your sexual responsiveness. Squeezing them

during sex produces more sensation in your genitals. Pumping them helps send sexual energy up through your energy-body.

Pelvic pumps

Now that you have isolated the love muscles and strengthened them, practise tipping your pelvis forward and backwards in time with pumping the muscles. This synchronized movement mimics the timing of thrusting during intercourse, and is a fabulous means of building your sexual fire during lovemaking, enhancing your erotic pleasure.

- Stand up with a straight back. If your neck is still stiff, let your head roll to one side, before slowly rolling it round backwards, to the other side, forwards and to the front. Roll it several times, gently stretching the muscles and releasing the tension with your breath.

- Bend your knees slightly so that you can move your hips easily. Check that the small of your back is loosened by circling your sacrum and tracing figures-of-eight with your hips.
- Breathe in as your pelvis tips forward. Squeeze the muscles around your anus upwards and hold these muscles as you hold your breath for a moment. Tuck your chin in towards your neck, lengthening the muscles at the back of the neck.
- As you breathe out, release the pelvic floor muscles, let your pelvis rock backwards (with the buttocks facing backwards) and release your chin.
- Breathe in again, rocking your hips forward and tucking your chin in. Keep up this pelvic rocking for some time, squeezing the love muscles with every inhalation.
- You can add an 'Ah' to the exhalation to emphasize a whole-body release as you relax your love muscles.

Pelvic rocking

In Tantra, learning how to direct your breath is the secret to discovering how to move energy through your body. The aim of this exercise is to synchronize your breathing with your partner, using visualization to imagine your energy rising through your energy centres at the same time. Combining this with pelvic rocking gives you a taste of the delights of Tantric sex.

- Sit cross-legged before your partner. As you both breathe in together, fall into a slow, deep rhythm of breathing – the man follows the woman's pace of breathing. Slow it down if your partner is struggling to keep up.
- When your joint breathing has established a natural rhythm, close your eyes and focus on visualizing the movement of breath up from your tailbone, through the centre of your body and up to your heart.
- Now imagine that you are drawing up the breath through your genitals into your pelvis. As you breathe

in, draw the energy into your pelvis. As you exhale, let it go back out through your genitals.

- When you have established this pattern, introduce a gentle forward-tilt of the hips (with genitals facing downwards) as you breathe in, and then tilt backwards (with genitals facing towards each other) as you breathe out. Continue breathing and rocking your pelvises together.

- Move into the classic Tantra posture of yab-yom, where the woman sits on her partner's lap with her legs wrapped around him.

- Practise circular breathing between you. To bring awakened erotic energy up through your spine toward your heart, start by imagining that you are drawing in your breath through your genitals as you gently rock your waist backwards (with genitals forwards), visualizing the energy climbing up to your heart. Send your out-breath from your heart to his as you rock your pelvis forwards. He breathes in deeply to receive this offering in his heart, then on the out-breath he sends the breath out through his genitals and into your genitals. Receive his outpouring through your vulva – inhale through your vagina as he exhales through his genitals. Breathe out through your heart, as he inhales your breath through his heart and sends it down to his pelvis and out through his penis.

- Maintain this cycling of sexual energy between heart and sex for many minutes, building up a heady state of arousal. You might be able to have an orgasm without genital stimulation just through rocking, squeezing and breathing.

Variation

You can both use hand gestures to demonstrate to your partner where your breath is located as it moves through your body. As you draw your breath from your genitals upwards through your body, you trace the path of your breath with your hand, opening your palm at your heart as you offer your lover your love and sexual energy *(see also Offering the lotus, page 94)*.

Pelvic rocking with the love-muscle squeeze

The following exercise combines the love-muscle squeeze with pelvic rocking during lovemaking. This intensifies the pleasure of thrusting during intercourse, especially for those who find it difficult to build up enough sexual excitement in order to reach orgasm.

Movement, breath and vocalization all improve your sexual vitality. In this powerful exercise you combine all three to enhance your sexual responsiveness. You generate sexual arousal through rhythmic movements, using your breath and visualization to raise the energy from your sexual centre and draw it upwards. This is essential for the experience of expanded orgasm, where the release of your sexual energy spreads through your whole body, sometimes shooting out through the top of your head.

- Sit comfortably facing your lover, with your legs loosely crossed. You can sit close together by both resting your right knee on your partner's left one.

169

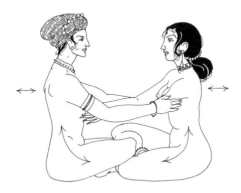

- Together, breathe in slowly and deeply at the same time, harmonizing your breathing. The woman usually sets the pace, but if her breathing is rapid and shallow the man breathes more slowly until she adapts. When your joint breathing has established a slow, easy rhythm, close your eyes and focus on visualizing the movement of breath through the energy channels up your spine.

- Both of you inhale together, imagining that you are pulling your breath in through your genitals at the base of your spine. As you release your breath, visualize it coming back out through your genitals. Breathe like this for several minutes as your sexual energy builds.

- Once you have established this pattern, continue breathing in this way and introduce a gentle forward-tilt of the pelvis (with genitals facing downwards) as you breathe in. Then tilt backward (with genitals facing towards each other) as you breathe out. As you breathe in, squeeze the love muscles around your genitals and anus. Release as you breathe out. This increases your sexual fire.

- Let the breath move upwards, in stages, through your hips, chest and head. With every inhalation bring your hips forward, and with every exhalation, tilt your hips backward. This moves energy through your sexual centre, your heart and towards the crown of your head.

- After several minutes of rocking your pelvis and squeezing the pelvic floor muscles, both of you imagine that you are drawing up your breath to the crown of your head. This prepares the way for energy to shoot

171

upwards. In Tantra the crown of the head, rather than the genitals, is regarded as the site of sexual bliss.

- When you feel that your breathing and energy is flowing, the woman moves into a sexual posture, sitting on the man's lap with her legs wrapped around his waist. Start to alternate your breathing as described in *Touching each other's hearts (Step 2, page 87):* to recap, the woman holds her breath while her partner exhales. Then when he next inhales, she exhales, so that he is breathing in her out-breath. She also holds her pelvis still while pausing and holding her breath. Once she starts moving her pelvis, both of you will be tilting back and forward simultaneously.

- As in *Pelvic rocking (see page 166),* the man inhales the woman's breath through his heart, sending it downwards and out through his penis. The woman imagines that she inhales through her vulva as he exhales through his genitals. This creates a circle of loving connection between you.

- If you sit in the man's lap, you can bring his penis inside you and continue the pelvic rocking and sexual breathing to rapidly intensify sexual arousal. Relax into your excitement. Let it build.

- Continue with sexual breathing, circling your breath between you through your hearts and genitals. Open to bliss.

Free your pelvis when you're turned off

If you don't feel satisfied with your sex life, it's likely that you have closed down the energy in your pelvis, or that there is some muscular tension and holding. The first thing to do is to shake out tension, mobilize your pelvis and get the energy moving into your sexual centre. You can do this through dance *(see pages 104, 106)* – find some dynamic, rhythmic music to shake in time to, shaking your pelvis vigorously and letting that shaking spread out into a fine trembling throughout your body. By opening your pelvis to movement, you open yourself to pleasure.

Another technique is to manipulate your pelvis while

lying on your back. This mobilizes pelvic energy, which can be particularly helpful if you feel numb or insensitive to sensual pleasure. You can do this on your own or together with your lover, lying side by side.

- Make yourself comfortable on your back, lying on a thick quilt. Bend your knees in order to let the small of your back rest on the floor. Lengthen your neck, relaxing your jaw, shoulders and hands. Make sure that your shoulders are not crunched up, and that your neck is not straining when you raise your pelvis off the floor.
- Breathe deeply to release stress or strain anywhere in your body. When you feel relaxed, lift your buttocks slightly, taking your weight on your feet and knees in order to gently shake your pelvis. Shake until your pelvis feels alive.
- Once you feel that your body is alive, stop moving and concentrate on the subtle sensations that arise in your pelvis. Encourage these vibrations to spread up your body.

Emotional wellbeing, sexual healing

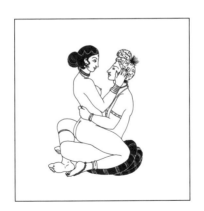

Emotional wellbeing means letting go of harmful emotional patterns in your relationship so that love can flourish. For good Tantric sex, you need to access the energy of love in your heart centre so your sexual energy can flow. Opening to love is a prerequisite to sexual bliss; if your heart is closed for any reason, the possibilities of love entering you are restricted.

Relationships tend to be full of conflict and misunderstanding. In Tantra, however, you can see these as missed opportunities to understand each other and grow. This Step explores how couples can be out of balance – both psychologically and energetically – and suggests strategies for reconnecting and rebalancing. Step 4 taught you how to awaken your sexual passion, but if you haven't been able to reach states of ecstasy because of emotional problems between you, this Step makes suggestions for clearing them. If you are feeling closed you will be shut down sexually as well. To revivify your sexual desire, you need to heal emotionally. Issues of sexual identity, power play and communication need to be addressed so that your sexual play is rich enough to be used as a basis for spiritual growth.

Emotional healing

The emotional texture of your inner world affects how you experience, connect with and relate to others. The levels of intimacy that each of you are comfortable with is often very different, because the emotional climate of your relationship is influenced by the climate of your family life when you were growing up. Some people will have had a warm, loving and tactile upbringing, while others may have felt isolated and lonely from an early age. Emotional distance in a relationship generally results from insufficient emotional recognition in the early years of life, or because as a child you closed off intense feelings when they threatened to overwhelm you. Introverted people may appear comfortable living in a cool, cut-off, emotionally shut-down environment, as it feels safer. Chaotic people may feel comfortable creating frequent emotional crises, because this is familiar to them from their early family environment.

Recognizing the positive and negative

You can help harmonize and balance the differences between you and your partner if you recognize that positive and negative emotions, such as pleasure and pain, are two different aspects of one energy. Both of you may be expressing a similar emotional intensity, but showing it in different ways. For instance, just as much energy may be invested in keeping away intimacy as in expressing the desire for intimacy. Whatever your feelings, it is vital to acknowledge their power, because they are also responsible for animating you. If you emote, you feel alive.

Emotional healing means ...

Getting some distance from emotional pain by not brooding on feelings

Loss and grief are part of most individuals' past experience, but holding onto your wounding tends to solidify it, trapping you in the past and distorting your present relationship. Engage in your current relationship without denying the damage from past experience. Choose to let it go, and allow the positive aspects of your life to refresh and nurture you.

Dropping your stance of inner conflict

By no longer judging emotions as bad, they lose some of their hold over you. Developing a healthy emotional attitude involves dropping your emotional posture – whether it is fear or a tendency to smother.

Reawakening your lust for life

When you are deeply in touch with your sexual being, you experience the vitality and energy that arise when your sexual power is unleashed. You can use this erotic energy to feel more dynamic and satisfied with life.

How to fall in love again

Sexuality is a dynamic expression of your psyche; it's a state of consciousness more than a biological drive. It enriches your relationships and your life. Some lovers, however, fall out of love. Over time, they fall away from one another instead of finding increased intimacy and a more fulfilling sexual connection. If you lose your desire, you can make a decision to turn yourself on again. Whether you are turned on or not is in your own hands, not those of your lover. Although it does help if your lover is feeling warm and sexually exploratory, the key to your sexuality is you, regardless of what's going on in your relationship. Knowing this helps you to recentre yourself.

Experience yourself as the source of your own pleasure and take responsibility for your own fulfilment.

Support each other in discovering your own desires; find ways of relating that are more sensual than sexual. For example, it might be more appropriate to go to jive classes together rather than focus on what's happening in bed! Exercises can be used only as long as they're useful – and then left behind.

This exercise is a good turning-on technique that you can use as a starting point to reawaken your desire. It can have a powerful, revitalizing effect upon you.

- Feel your sexual energy emanating from your pelvis. Sense it penetrating your whole body. Revel in the sensuality of your body. You are an erotic being.
- Imagine an intense inner heat at the core of your being. Visualize this heat as a red fire that permeates your body. Feel your sexual energy enlivening you. Enjoy your lust for life.
- Feel your sexual being and sexual power. Don't think it, feel it.
- As you go about your daily life, allow this sexual energy to be in your awareness. Don't cut off from

it, judging it inappropriate, embarrassing or distracting. Sexuality is your true nature. Allow it to colour
your interactions with warmth, passion and a sexual
presence.

Freeing your mind

Emotions are no more real than your thoughts. Regard
them as bodily reactions to your mind – when you feel
anxious, your body will be tense and contracted; if you
feel angry or are withdrawn from your partner, your
body will mirror the negativity of your thoughts by
tensing up or expressing agitated movement.

It's important to identify your negative emotions
about your partner in order to heal them. Usually our
mind runs the scripts of our relationships, forcing them
along familiar lines. If we get stuck in our minds, we re-
run old wounds or rehearse for future disappointments.
Our thoughts can generate discontent, anger and
resentment. Such negative emotions are likely to be
coming from your false self (the one that identifies with

your negative thoughts) rather than your authentic self (the part of you that is guided by your heart). Those lucky people who are in touch with their true nature much of the time say that this state is characterized by feelings of contentment, peace and joy. They describe their awareness as a pure, unmediated lovingness in which their attitude towards others is one of compassion, rather than blame or disappointment. When you feel compassionate, you can accept your partner's imperfections, along with your own.

In holding on to your wounds, you cling to the defensive character that you have created in response to pain. Past experiences hamper your openness by out-of-date responses conditioned by past experiences. So instead of expressing emotions such as fear, anger or coldness, recognize that they are manufactured by your mind and choose to drop them.

Healing a lack of love
by giving love

Your desperation for love can make you accept relation-ships in which there are only crumbs of love available, insufficient to nourish you. But before you jettison the relationship, check whether the problem is your own ability to give and receive love. If you don't feel suffi-ciently loved, try to focus on giving love rather than complaining about a sense of lack. If you feel unloved, the most usual response is to close down your heart so that it becomes even more difficult to receive any love from others. Consider the following.

- Loving others dissolves self-protective or defensive modes of being.
- Loving is the way to heal feelings of isolation, aban-donment or rejection. Grief and disappointment can leave you feeling depressed and lonely, bitter and mistrustful or critical and judgmental of others – all of which are expressions of a sense of alienation.

- To heal any wounding that has been creating barriers around your heart, open up again to the existence of love.

Healing a fear of intimacy through constancy

Closeness paradoxically causes fear because sharing our lives with another makes us all too aware of the likelihood of future loss. Many couples try to alleviate such feelings by forging a strong dependency that provides emotional security for one another. However, apparent closeness can cause its own problems as any differences may have to be suppressed. Not communicating with honesty is the surest way to prevent real intimacy developing, and we need deep intimacy in order to explore our full sexual potential *(see the Authentic communication exercises in Step 2, page 66)*. It's in a relationship where both individuals are differentiated that they can choose to be together through desire, rather than emotional neediness.

Think how the constancy of your relationship helps to heal a fear of intimacy. Relax into your relationship and develop faith in your lover and their fundamental integrity. In order to really trust each other, drop your lack of trust and suspicion. Possessiveness is a sign of fear rather than intimacy. It can be a strategy for creating a sense of safety – for example, re-creating relationships of dependency, like those you had with your parents.

The thought of merging your identities may be seductive, but this urge often manifests as possession; it's also difficult to be in a Tantric relationship unless you can feel fulfilled when you are separate, because the key to a growing relationship is to know yourself. A desire for merging might be a defence against pain and neglect, which need to be healed on your own. Your relationship can act as a supportive container while you do this, but ultimately it is up to you to heal your own wounds.

Open-heart meditation

Mature sexual love is created between two separate individuals overflowing with love. Opening the heart centre is crucial to deepening love and finding more intimacy. Through meditation, you can discover that your heart is a place of unconditional lovingness. Regular meditation helps you to drop your defences so you can respond to life in a receptive, spontaneous and open way, relating from your heart rather than your mind.

Practice the Open-heart meditation below, or try the Rosebud meditation *(page 97)* or Touching each other's hearts *(page 87)*.

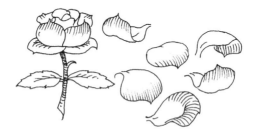

- Sit in meditation and let your breathing deepen and lengthen.
- Breathe into your heart area.
- Imagine your heart beating.
- Imagine your heart softening.
- Imagine your heart expanding.

Healing shame

Shame is based on a feeling of worthlessness – an internalized belief that you are not acceptable as you are, which creates a feeling of failure.

Think about the myriad of ways that children are shamed for just being themselves; what they say, what they do, how they behave, their perceptions and insights. They are often teased mercilessly, and consequently they may internalize a sense that they are not good enough as they are, unless they behave in the ways that their peers or parents wish. This underlying lack of self-esteem can be covered up with compensatory strategies that manifest as egotistic or shameless behaviour.

This can be the case when sex is filtered through pornographic fantasy or where sado-masochistic practices shape sexual relationships. While it might be potentially healing to explore taboos, there is the risk of reinforcing more destructive ways of relating. Exploring taboos needs to be done in a gentle, self-loving way. Because sexuality is associated with shame in our culture, sexual addiction might stem from deep feelings of shame, or a desperate need for love. Healing shame involves letting manipulation or power struggles fall away so that you can simply be yourself – without judging yourself, or worrying about the judgment of others.

Healing shame through self-love

In this exercise, what's most erotic is seeing the pleasure you take in your own body. It's not what your body looks like, but how you inhabit it that makes it appear sexy to the on-looker. Eroticism comes from living in, and enjoying, your own physical nature and the sensuality of life. It arises from enjoying the sexy fact that you are alive and that you have a body to give you pleasure.

- Strip off slowly, as performing a striptease for your partner. He or she says what he likes about your body as you slowly reveal each part of it. Stand before your lover in all your nakedness …
- As you reveal your body, ask your lover to express his or her delight. It is very important to hear your partner's appreciation of you – many couples don't get the chance to hear compliments often enough.
- Concentrate on your own experience rather than imagining what your partner might be thinking. Enjoy your bodily sensations as you remove each garment slowly and sensually.

A visualization for letting go of trauma and shame

If you have been humiliated as a child or sexually traumatized you may need to return to an inviolate state of innocence in order to respond to your partner according to what is happening in the present moment, without all your emotional baggage from the past. You can do this through dissolving the guilt and shame learnt as a consequence of your earliest experiences.

This meditation is for those who feel stuck in sadness and negativity, and can't let in joy and bliss. Emotional pain may have formed a cloud-like 'pain-body', blighting the vitality of your being. Picture your suffering as an energetic mass of pain that represents past traumatic experiences or emotional difficulties that have cramped emotional flexibility and created compensations, distortions or emotional withholding. This psychological tension will be mirrored by physical tension in your body. Picturing your emotional pain as a pain-body may help you to dissolve it through this healing meditation.

- Let healing white light cleanse your body of the residue of painful and sad memories stored in your tissues. As you imagine white light washing through

you, imagine a dark cloud of negativity being washed
out and dispersing into the stream of white light.

- As the toxicity of abuse and shame is released from
your cells, your being is left cleansed and vibrant.

Healing a lack of confidence
through dignity

Instead of complaining about how your partner doesn't
support you or why they won't give you what you
believe you want, approach them with a sense of your
own dignity, worth and the fullness of your experience.

Heal self-doubt through cultivating a sense of
presence. The meditations in Step 1 are very useful
for helping you develop this capacity to affirm your
inner being – see the affirmations on loving your body
(pages 5, 35). This five-minute mantra will help pick you
up during those moments when you feel insecure or
unattractive.

Beauty is ...

I am my essential nature. I can shine.

My body has beauty. It gives me pleasure.

I thank my body for everything that it does.

Releasing negative emotions

If you have become stuck in a familiar pattern of emotional wounding (such as crying or getting angry again and again) expressing your emotions is not always positive. Continually expressing negative emotions when they are no longer productive shapes your internal life. Instead, learn to see emotions as just an energy charge, so that love and hate are merely different expressions of intense energy. Both love and hate

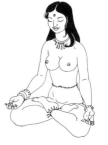

bind you into a relationship with your partner, regardless of the form your emotions take. Seen in this way,
you can make a choice about how you wish to express
your emotions. Do you want to be attached through
love, or through negativity? The exercise below will
help you get more clarity on your feelings.

Writing off negativity

In this ritual, you try to create a gap between experiencing your emotions and reacting to them by writing them
down. This gap is a period of time during which a
deeper awareness can enter – you can try to evaluate the
appropriateness of your emotions, and make choices
about how you want to act on them. In the process of
evaluation, consider the effects that your response will
have on your partner. Then use compassionate awareness to heal your relationship. Through regular meditation practice, you can let go of blaming your partner.

• Start by thinking about all the grudges and resentments

you have about your partner. List all of the ways that you feel they have hurt you or let you down. What are the reasons, and why?

- Now add to your list: note all the emotional responses that you feel limit you and hold you back. List your fear, resentment, envy, sloth, small-mindedness, lack of generosity … anything and everything.

- By transferring all your grudges and negativities to paper, you begin to clear your mind. Now carefully light a match and slowly hold it to the paper. Burn the bad and let go as you watch each line burning. Imagine the fire of your passionate awareness incinerate every one.

- Burn the list. Let go of the resentments as you watch the paper burning. Imagine that this flame is inside your body, cleansing you of toxic emotions. Imagine it in your belly, rising up through your body and into your head. Let it consume your frustration, discontent or resentment. When the page has burned away, you will have fully let go of everything written upon it.

- Now sit in front of your partner. Feel your love. Gaze at him or her with soft eyes full of loving kindness.

Allow your love to dissolve any resentment or hurt that you have been holding on to. Resentment hurts you more than anyone else, so let go of it.

- Realize that there is nothing to forgive. Try to let go of anything your lover has said or done to hurt you, whether intentionally or not. Let go in this very moment. Experience your mutual forgiveness as a bridge that links your two hearts.

- From a position of compassion you can see that anything hurtful someone does is inevitably the result of his or her own wounding or pain.

- With every breath, feel the similarity between you and send out love. Sit gazing at each other for several minutes, resting in the atmosphere of compassion. You are two souls trying to do the best you can.

Allowing the positive

Sometimes we don't believe that we can have what we want, or are unable to accept the good things on offer in life. When your relationship feels stuck, the way through it is to allow the positive.

- Focus on what you have rather than on what appears to be lacking.
- When your mind goes to your perception of what is lacking, pull it up and instead concentrate on the good things that you experience when you're together. Focus on the warmth, closeness and companionship; the understanding, the playful times, the laughter. Recall the pleasures of lovemaking. Let the memories of these joyful times warm you and nourish your spirit.

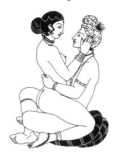

Healing criticism: still your mind

Most people get irritated by things about each other. Yet blaming others for the way that they are implies that you are not taking responsibility for yourself and your own behaviour.

It is important to learn to detach from criticism and blame, which is a consequence of our overly busy minds. Blaming and complaining are signs of passive aggression rather than taking charge of your own contribution to the problem. Are you behaving in a way that shows your better qualities or that brings out the best in your partner? The golden rule is to always look at your own behaviour first – after all, you can only change yourself. These tips help you tune out habitual negative thinking.

- Turn off the analytical, critical function of your mind. Be still. Simply be.
- Let go of your doubt, distrust or suspicion towards others.

- Let go of competition and envy. Bless others for what they have.
- Drop your feelings of arrogance and superiority, or shame and self-consciousness.
- Stop denigrating. Denigrating others is usually associated with a deep (sometimes unconscious) belief that you are not okay yourself.

Converting irritation through loving kindness

This exercise encourages you to take responsibility for your emotions rather than blame your partner for failing to do what you want. It clears away the petty irritations that can create resentment and blocks to intimacy, fostering greater trust and understanding.

- When you feel irritability arise, send out loving kindness toward your partner and compassion towards them for whatever deficiencies or habits irritate you.

- Improvise a short meditation in which you focus on feeling compassion toward your own efforts to improve the relationship, as well as the efforts of your lover.

Healing communication through active listening

To listen and be listened to is essential in any partnership. Active listening is when you focus all your attention on your partner as he or she tries to articulate their concerns.

Actively listening to your partner means that you really hear what they are saying without rushing in to comment, analyze or defend yourself – or to change the subject. These are all strategies for not wanting to listen. This exercise helps you to feel heard, even if your sentiments are not always understood or agreed with.

- It may be that you are trying to get your own point across without thinking about the listener's perspective. To reach them, be aware of their responses. If your partner refuses to listen to anything you say, you may have to let them speak first so that they feel heard – then they might be able to drop their own agenda and actually take a turn listening to you.

- Whenever your relationship is under strain, marriage guidance counsellors recommend having fifteen minutes each to talk, without comment or interruption. This is an essential relationship skill that trains you to have the confidence to speak about whatever is on your mind, as well as practising actively listening.

Healing a lack of connection: become a witness

If you want to feel more connected to your partner, you may have to stop trying so hard. You don't need to share your partner's troubles or try to fix their problems. Instead of trying to make them feel better or attempting to analyse their behaviour, try to attune yourself to their energy. This means sensing the quality of their being;

who they really are underneath all their preoccupations and habits.

A witness sees deeply into the other person – perceiving their essence rather than relating to their sometimes-unpleasant modes of behaving. The previous Active listening exercise helps you to be more of an observer, rather than rushing to cut through your partner's monologue with your reactions. To become a witness to your partner's internal processes, aim to observe them without explaining away or judging what they are saying.

Let go of your own preconceptions about what is going on in their minds.

- Simply sit together for twenty minutes.
- Look at your lover without wavering. Hold him or her in your gaze, so that they literally feel held by your regard.
- Focus all your attention on being aware of your partner. Try to experience them as they experience themselves. Be aware of the quality of the core energy they are emanating.

Healing disillusionment:
let go of your illusions

Disillusionment means having to dissolve your illusions about yourself and your relationship.

In the past, you had ideas (illusions) about who you are, and who your partner is and how your relationship operates. This five-minute visualization helps you focus on the heart of your relationship rather than your ideas about how it should be.

• Imagine all your assumptions and fantasies about your partner dissolving. Visualize this as a flame that touches your disillusion.

• Let the heat of the flame melt away the tissues of your hopes and desires. Let it burn away any fantasies constructed around your relationship, revealing its essential core – the dance of energy between you.

Fire meditation for clearing obstructions

Fire has long been used by Tantrics to burn away blocks in your energy-body. When energy moves through your body, it is easier to harness it to your spiritual development.

- Stand with your spine straight and your feet planted on the floor, in line with your shoulders. Plant your legs on the ground as if you are sending roots down into the earth, through your feet.
- Let the fire take you over. Move or dance as that flame

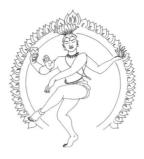

consumes your body. Imagine the fiery energy of the red flame entering your pelvis. Let it burn away any sexual wounding or tension. As you feel clearer, let the flame ignite and feed your sexual energy and power.

- After a few minutes, imagine the flame climbing higher towards your navel. Your belly and abdomen are transformed into a crucible in which any creative blocks are fired with new energy. Imagine the fire clearing away the old as it climbs up to the area of your solar plexus.

- When the flame licks at the inside of your chest, let it burn away any emotional wounds you are holding in your heart. Let it cleanse and open your heart centre.

- In the area of your throat, imagine that the fire burns away any blocks to self-expression and communication.

- The flames create focus and clarity as they consume your third-eye area, burning out old redundant ways of viewing the world and other people.

- As the flames subside, imagine that you feel cleansed and renewed, awash with feelings of contentment, clarity and energy.

- Imagine that you are open and full of passion for life, energized and creatively stimulated. As the heat subsides, welcome a sense of space, vision and clarity. Enjoy this awareness of greater openness and clearer communication.
- Bask in a brilliant sense of your own presence and empowerment. Feel sexually cleansed and renewed. Celebrate your passion for life.

Healing need through caring for yourself

When you feel genuinely connected with your lover, your sexual energy flows with a sense of vitality, abundance and sensual pleasure. However, if you are overly needy of others, you may be using sex to try to connect. This can be the basis of a sexual addiction in which over-involvement with others distracts you from your own emotional issues. When you are busy looking after the needs of others, you don't feel your own grief, loneliness or anxiety. Such issues need to be sorted out before you can start exploring your sexual potential.

This is a simple but radical visualization that can be quite startling, and shocks you into letting go of your state of emotional neediness. You realize that your expectations of your partner to assuage your feelings may be unrealistic, overwhelming or even frightening to them.

- Imagine what it would be like to be your partner, staring into the bottomless pit of your own needs.
- Imagine what it would feel like if it were your responsibility to try to meet those needs.

Healing drama or crisis through centring yourself

Take responsibility for clearing your own negative emotions and centring yourself, so that you don't create disharmony through your own inner chaos. Negative feelings need to be released in order to prevent physical holding and emotional withholding. Anger and resentment will prevent the possibility of rising above your negativity.

However, if you take responsibility for your own emotional state, you can recognize that anger and resentment are of no benefit to anyone.

- Use this martial arts posture: centre yourself by standing with your feet hip-distance apart, knees slightly bent and back straight, to align your spine and allow energy to flow easily.
- Close your eyes and take a few minutes to go inside yourself, concentrating on your breathing. Focus on your inhalation and exhalation, and observe the rhythm of your own breathing. Allow it to become longer and slower.
- As you inhale, imagine that your breath is travelling down to your tailbone at the base of your spine. As you exhale, imagine it moving back up your spine to exit through your lungs.
- Push out the breath from your belly with a 'hah' sound. Use each out-breath to forcibly expel your

frustration, irritation or anger. Throw off resentment, harsh judgments or self-protective withdrawal. Release your impulse to wound your partner in retaliation for your own wounding. By expelling all these aggressive states, you release your anger and return to a calm state of 'being'.

Healing your power-struggle

If you are still trying to change each other, then it's likely that you are both locked in a power-struggle. Resolving the struggle involves creating a complementary balance within the relationship by accepting your differences as complementing each other.

So often we become stuck in polarized positions; men acting out their phallic energy, while women passively surrender. Or, women denigrate their men for their inadequacies. We can heal this polarity by acknowledging that all of us have both male and female aspects – Tantra involves getting in touch with your inner man or woman. In lovemaking you weave together your own male and female energies, merging your sexually active and receptive drives, your lust and your love, your awareness and your compassion. Through using breathing and visualizations that connect your sexual energy with your heart and wisdom centres, your inner man and woman begin to make love with each other – by exchanging energy.

Kissing is symbolic of the alchemical mixing of male and female principles in which your energies are exchanged and merged. Through the exchange of sexual energies during kissing, the polarity between you is bridged and the power-struggle resolved.

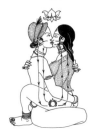

- As you kiss, drink in the essence of your partner as your saliva mingles. Imagine that as you imbibe their mouth juices you are absorbing their qualities, whether passionate and fiery or cool and still.
- Find a place of passionate stillness in the midst of your kiss.

Healing resentment and suffering through forgiveness

In order to demolish unhelpful defences it is necessary to let go of bitterness or resentment, and forgive those who have wounded you – whether this is your partner, an ex-lover or your parents. However, many people resist forgiveness because in some way this lets the guilty party off the hook. When someone has behaved unacceptably, they fear that their forgiveness gives the perpetrators subtle permission to repeat their bad behaviour. However, the only person who gets damaged by your constant bitterness is you. In forgiving the other person, you free yourself from your own bad feelings and antagonism. Once forgiveness melts your emotional armouring, you can open to the free flow of energy through your body once again.

In this meditation, you see another's struggle for happiness, and acknowledge that they are fundamentally just like you. Look on the ways in which they express their difficulties in life with an attitude of compassion. Bear in mind that they are doing the best they can, just as you are trying to do your best to find happiness. Feel this compassion filling your heart with warm, loving feelings.

- With every exhalation, send out waves of compassion. Transmit vitality and healing to your partner. With your out-breath, send the thought, 'may you be free of suffering'.
- Close the meditation with a warm, loving embrace.

If your relationship is loving, it can offer mutual healing on physical, emotional and soul levels. You can embrace emotional distress or mental anguish in a spirit of love. This is part of the work of deepening your relationship to reach profound levels of intimacy.

A meditation for compassion

Compassion encompasses gentleness, kindness and understanding. Do you feel compassionate towards those who are closest to you? Toward acquaintances? Do you value them as much as you value yourself? Do you value yourself as much as you value others?

Recognizing the effect of your actions on others results in the realization that it is a priority to live your life with integrity. It is important not to add to the collective pool of suffering by doing anything that might intentionally or inadvertently harm others. Dedicate your life to helping others in whatever ways you can.

The key Buddhist practice of taking on other's pain is a real challenge to your usual strategy of trying to avoid anything that might potentially cause suffering. This is a radically different way of thinking about suffering; instead of trying to avoid emotional pain at all costs, you work on developing a deep compassion towards yourself and others. Through an acceptance of suffering, you realize that you can carry the difficulties of others. You don't need to be afraid of it. You can support others by absorbing their suffering and letting their angst flow through you as energy. If you view it as pure energy, you won't get stuck with holding onto any problems. You will discover that you can relieve them of their burden without harming yourself.

Use this meditation to convert trivial irritations into loving kindness toward your partner and dissolve the separation between you both. See yourselves as fellow travellers struggling through life. You are fundamentally the same as every other human being on the planet.

- Sit comfortably facing your partner. Close your eyes and bring your attention to your own breath. Let it settle into a slow, gentle rhythm as you imagine your lungs filling with air and emptying.

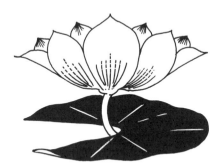

- Picture your partner being upset. See them in your mind's eye. Imagine that your partner is sitting in front of you in all their vulnerability and unhappiness.
- As you breathe in, you take on all their anxiety, pain and suffering in order to relieve them of their burden. With your out-breath, send them compassionate love.
- With every inhalation, keep taking in their distress and with every exhalation bathe them in love. You will discover that it is easy for you to take on their troubles. You can dissolve their pain in the softness and love of your compassionate heart.

215

A meditation for healing suffering: surrender to change

If you consider that suffering is the energy-pattern of a closed heart, you can see that suffering can have a positive aspect – but you will be unaware of it when you're immersed in emotional pain. Suffering is largely created through desire and need. Through the frustration that life brings, your habitual ways of defining yourself are weakened. Your identity can crack apart. If you can remain aware as you surrender to the process of seeming to fall apart, the unexpected benefit is that a different quality of being and perception begins to emerge.

The art of accepting change is to surrender to whatever is happening, regardless of your fears and anxieties about it. Remaining aware of your reactions and inner processes helps you to reach greater acceptance. We all have the capacity to love and to respond to love, no matter what damage we have endured.

- Lie in the corpse posture, fully relaxed *(see page 30).*

Close your eyes, and concentrate on your breathing.

- As you relax more deeply, imagine the whole of life as a vast ocean. Feel the water washing the underside of your body. Surrender to the movement of the waves.
- Let the water buffet you. Become aware of its strength and power, and feel confident that the sea will support you. Let the sea hold you.
- Relax. Float. Let the ocean carry you to its destination.

Sexual healing

If you suffer from the sexual problems described in medical parlance as 'dysfunctions', such as difficulty reaching orgasm, premature ejaculation or impotence, they are often due to emotional wounding and an inhibition of your sexual energy, which has resulted in physical and emotional tension. Tantra is perfect for sexual healing because of its stress on whole-body sensuality, loving connection and the use of breath and visualization to arouse yourself, in addition to the traditional pleasures of genital friction.

Your ability to appreciate what the present moment offers may be damaged by past wounds from invasions, rejections and expectations. Cutting off and emotional distance may be the residue of difficult past sexual experiences *(see page 177)*. Distressing emotions evoked by body memories can arise during sex. I think it's most healing if you can accept the intrusion of these old emotions into the present and remain in your beloved's arms while you try to detach from your upset. Your body might be closed down, closed off to enjoyment, withholding from giving.

If it is hard to receive sexual pleasure because you feel you can't cope with the difficult feelings that arise, try not to push it away. Experiment with more pleasure, more regularly (little and often) until you feel receptive. The pleasure itself will soften your defences and invite an expansion of energy from your core. Deep healing restores your sexuality and encourages a positive sense of self.

In healing sexual difficulties, it is also important to explore the emotional and soulful qualities of sex as well as the technical aspects. In this way, you can bring the sacred back into the bedroom.

A healing meditation for sexual wounding

This meditation is best practised when you are being held by your lover. He or she lies with you, harmonizing his/her breathing with yours and sensing your inner emotional state.

- Relax with meditation *(see page 35)*, going inside yourself and stilling your mind. Go into your body. Relax and release any tension.
- Imagine that the surface of your body has become permeable, visualizing molecules dancing both in and around your body. Open up to the molecules outside your body. Open up to your partner. As a pair, open

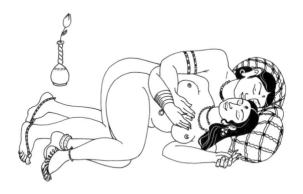

to the world outside the two of you.

- Sense where in your body you might still be holding deep tension. Send your attention to any site of holding and, as you breathe out, imagine that you are letting go of this tension. Your partner can place their hand over this area, supporting you as you try to dissolve any bodily armouring and release any resistance to healing. Common areas to work with are the shoulders, and neck, the small of the back, the womb and the groin.

Healing difficulty with orgasm

For women, difficulty releasing sexual energy in orgasm may be the result of inadequate clitoral stimulation or poor lovemaking techniques, insufficient intimacy, or the scars of anxiety and emotional wounding.

These issues may be as much energetic or emotional as physiological. Negative body memories can create these problems. If you are carrying a lot of physical tension, you need to go back to the exercises in Step 1 to relax, still your mind and cleanse and revitalize your energy-body *(see pages 6, 42, 46)*. Then you may need to follow the suggestions in Step 2 about focusing on love and connection, affirming the heart of your relationship rather than worrying about sex not working *(see pages 66, 73)*.

Sexual problems, such as an inability to orgasm, may be the result of inadequate genital stimulation. However, difficulty with orgasm, impotence or prema-ture ejaculation may also be the result of blocked energy. Tantra teaches you how to build up your sexual energy and concentrate on increasing your own sexual arousal, rather than relying on your partner to do it all for you – which is a good idea if they're not a particularly skilled or adventurous lover. You can then embark on the journey of sexual exploration together. Through the healing dance of real connection, sexual problems get replaced by sexual communion. Good sex creates energy – it doesn't deplete it.

Healing premature ejaculation

Generally, men need to learn to defer their gratification. This book shows you how to respond to more subtle sensual touch and extend your pleasure beyond genital gratification – to stop going for the big 'O', and to separate coming from ejaculation so that you can experience multiple orgasms instead of one short one. Ejaculation signals the dispersal of sexual excitement and the end of pleasure. Wouldn't you like to learn how to prolong enjoyment for yourself and your partner – for as long as possible? See the exercises in Step 6 *(pages 262–268)*.

Healing difficulties with erection

For men, physiological changes to do with ageing, ill-health or an underlying lack of self-esteem compounded by fear of failure may cause difficulties with sustaining an erection. Tantric techniques can help repair problem areas by shifting the focus to what works, then building upon positive experiences. Sexual problems may reflect a difficulty surrendering to sexual energy, or allowing excitement to build up and be contained within your body without immediately dissipating the charge. For instance, this may be the source of the problem for men who come after very little genital contact or for women who cannot sustain arousal in order to build toward orgasm. The exercise below can help heal erection difficulties, because it encourages genital pleasure rather than intercourse.

Soft-erection sex

In Tantra, male and female energy is considered complementary – the energy exchange that occurs via the genitals during sex is vital for balancing you and your partner. In this exercise, a soft erection is a bonus because it helps you focus on the subtle sensations that arise when you merely join your genitals together, rather than the more familiar pleasures of genital friction.

- Your partner can encourage your penis to engorge with blood by creating a ring with her finger at the base of your penis, or stimulating your genitals with her mouth.
- For soft penetration, rub your penis around your lover's pearl (clitoris). When it becomes more erect, rub it into the entrance of the vagina, swirling around the entrance and back up to circle the pearl.
- To enter her vagina when soft, massage her vulva with your soft penis, and then guide the head of it into the entrance of her vagina, using your two fingers. This

feels particularly nice while sitting upright with your backs straight, if you can manage it. Otherwise, try the scissors position, where you both lie on your side facing each other, with the man's hips between his partner's open legs, so that he can access her vagina easily.

- The man focuses on using his penis to transmit loving feelings, rather than using it as an instrument for genital stimulation. Concentrate all your loving and sexual feelings into your penis, and send them into your lover's vagina. You may like to visualize this as a fiery, red energy, or as an abundant white liquid that pours all your good feelings into your partner.

- She can imagine this loving genital contact as nourishing, and a source of goodness.

- Alternate a state of total relaxation spreading from your genitals throughout your body, with squeezing your love muscles together, or using gentle stroking for pleasurable sensation anywhere on the body.

A daily meditation from the heart

To ensure your emotional wellbeing and a loving sexual connection try this meditation on a daily basis. It is also perfect before any of the healing exercises discussed in this chapter. Use it whenever you need healing: sexual, emotional and spiritual.

Imagine your body wrapped in a ball of golden light, like a cocoon. Then imagine a translucent pink light, the soft colour of rose quartz crystal, in the heart area of your chest, which gradually permeates your whole body and expands to colour the golden ball pink. Spend several minutes a day doing this meditation – while sitting quietly or lying down in a relaxed position. If you are doing it with your partner, you can visualize the cocoon around both of you.

STEP SIX

Sex
secrets

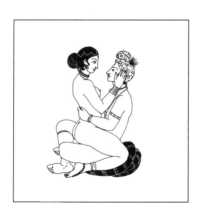

Even the most sexually confident people can pay more attention to sexual technique. There will always be some nuance that we haven't experienced before, and some response that takes us by surprise. After all, sex is the treasure at the heart of your relationship, the physical expression of your love. It's a sign of great love to try and explore the breadth and depths of your partner's sexual response so that together you can enjoy the great possibilities inherent in lovemaking.

There are a number of Tantric tips for making the most of sex, all of which are explained in this Step. To get the most out of these secrets, you need to take responsibility for your own pleasure first. Get yourself into a state of sexual aliveness and erotic excitement by whatever means works for you. Once you are making love it is up to you to ask for what you want during sex, and make sure you give your partner plenty of appreciative feedback about what you enjoy.

Although some of the Tantra exercises sound exotic, remember that simple things can be extremely aphrodisiac: just looking at each other or kissing is a big turn-on for most people. Holding hands is a favourite expression of closeness, and you can do this while meditating *(see page 35)*. Take time over sensual touch and slow stroking. Keep it simple: you can use basic tools, such as feathers and silken robes, but your best sex aids are your imagination and your love. With love, you can go a long way in sex; your feelings of love create a special quality of lovemaking.

Orgasm is another big turn-on. A positive frame of mind makes it easier to come, so get yourself into a sexy and confident mood for lovemaking. Men adore it when their partner has an orgasm – it validates men as sexual beings, making them feel great that they have helped their partner reach sexual satisfaction.

The best sex

The best sex is sex that brings you closer. The heart of Tantra is about enhancing intimacy, because the more you are attuned to each other, the more fulfilling sex will be. Below are three fundamental tips to consider before you begin making love.

1 Nurture your energy

The secret of Tantric sex is the art of dynamic relaxation. Your body should be relaxed before you make love, and your energy should be tended before embarking on lovemaking. If you use sex as a form of tension release, its possibilities might be reduced to a functional experience. You can use dance or a dynamic meditation such as that on page 104 to revitalize you when you are tired. Once your energy has been awakened you can relax into the sensual pleasures of simple touch.

2 Loving lovemaking

Make love from a place of connection. Whenever you are distracted or disengaged for any reason, keep returning your focus to a feeling of love between you and your partner. Feel at one with your lover. It helps you to merge if you imagine that you are one body – what they feel, you feel. Their pleasure is the same as your pleasure. Treat them as tenderly as you would like to be treated. Touch them with respect and love. The slower and more gentle your touch, the more subtle and rich your lover's sensual response.

3 Open-eyed sex
Deepen your level of intimacy during lovemaking by keeping your eyes open throughout sexual play. This simple but effective technique will keep your attention fully focused on your partner and absorbed in the energy being exchanged between you. To experience the increased closeness that gazing evokes, try to look into your partner's eyes throughout the whole lovemaking session. Soften your eyes, and gaze at them with love.

Foreplay

The best foreplay is spending time enjoying each other's company – sharing your day or having a heart-to-heart, so you feel connected on an emotional level. Foreplay can also mean relaxing together in a hot bubble bath, meditating together, doing yoga or dancing to music. Foreplay means entering the spirit of play. Enjoy creating your own private games and sensual adventures. Invent your own unique rituals to celebrate your relationship.

One of the simplest ways to get more out of foreplay and your sensual relationship is to cultivate being in the present. If you feel your mind taking over or your thoughts stray, bring your attention back to the bond between you, and focus on the quality of the sensations you're experiencing. There is no point in making comparisons between this occasion and a previous one, or this partner and a previous one. Let go of any difficult emotions of resentment or anger. Being in the present is a remarkably effective way to intensify your erotic pleasure.

Gazing and caressing

In this ritual approach to looking and touching, you enliven and sensitize your bodies through your gaze, caresses and sensual touch. Begin by sharing a meal or a glass of light wine together. Be playful. Pass a sip of liqueur from mouth to mouth; with your fingers, anoint your lover's lips and tongue with wine. When you are ready, move into the bedroom.

- Close the bedroom door and light a candle.
- Spend some time just looking at your partner, appreciating their love and support, their loyalty, their beauty. Share how much you cherish their body.
- Massage each other, or touch each other with gentle eroticism. Rest in a melting embrace, or lie together just breathing. Harmonize your breath in order to harmonize your beings.

Variation

Try using sensual touch to turn your lover on before you go out. This kind of foreplay will warm the woman up and keep both of you in a state of pleasurable anticipation. The waves of sexual energy that you feel while you're out act as a reminder of your erotic intention.

When you get home, you can make love.

You start with any of the sexy exercises in this book when you wake up in the morning. Allow sensual impressions to flood your being throughout the day, without embarrassment or discomfort. Relish the thought of getting home to your lover.

Use this as an opportunity to discover how sexual arousal can vitalize your energy, day and night. Sexual energy is not just about sexual desire; it's about your lust for life. Learn to arouse it and use it to enhance all areas of your life. Life is sexy!

Erotic kissing

Your tongue is important for creating an energy circuit, which transfers energy through your joined lips. When your tongues are intertwined or your breath mingles, the two of you come together as one.

This exercise helps you to feel the connection between the upper lip and the clitoris, and the upper lip and the tip of the penis. This energy circuit is at its most power-ful when both your genitals and tongues are connected, which is why kissing during intercourse is so intensely pleasurable. Because these erogenous zones – the upper lips and genitals – are linked, pleasuring any one of them makes the others more sensitive.

- While your partner nibbles and sucks your upper lip, you nibble his lower lip.
- While stimulating your lip, he caresses your nipple with one hand and your clitoris with the other. Alternatively, you can stroke your own clitoris to give him a free hand for other stimulation. The clitoris corresponds to the head of his penis so you can rub that area gently, using saliva or natural yoghurt to lubricate.

Enchantment

To increase sexual sensitivity and lengthen arousal, focus on body sensuality. Slow touch builds erotic pleasure more completely and surely than genital stimulation. It enables partners to synchronize their levels of desire and arousal, giving you the time to sensitize different parts of the body.

- Start with slow breathing, harmonizing your breathing with one other.
- Put all your attention in your fingertips to build arousal, being as subtle and delicate as you can. Caress each other's bodies with feathers, breath, fingertips, mouth and tongue. Often, women need to have their whole body touched, appreciated and pleasured before you zero in on genital stimulation. Men like having their penis and scrotum acknowledged before you move your hands up their abdomen and down their thighs to stroke the rest of their body.
- Sexual energy spreads through your body when you caress less obvious erogenous zones, such as the neck, earlobes, the delicate areas along the waist, the wrist, behind the knees, the inner thighs and breasts.
- To increase your sexual sensitivity you need to

contain this arousal, letting it enliven your body and fire your sexual passion without hurrying on to the next stage. Spend time basking in your heightened sexual responsiveness, appreciating the experience for itself rather than wanting to scratch your sexual itch.

Touching and tasting

In the following exercises you use your fingers and tongue to pleasure each other into a state of heightened arousal, or to orgasm. If you explore your lover's anatomy intimately through touch – stroking and sucking your lover's juices – you gather more insight on how to pleasure each other during sex.

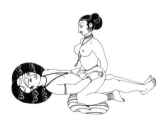

Breast massage

Breasts are associated with the heart and love, so massaging them helps activate loving nurturing emotions in both men and women. The heart centre is located between the breasts, and this is the area that you focus on during meditation to activate your love and infuse your sexual activity with love.

- Touch the heart region between your lover's breasts, stroking it delicately. Blow on the chest, drawing your fingertips or eyelashes over the skin as you move toward the breasts.
- Uncover your lover's breasts slowly and tenderly. Give him or her some appreciative feedback. You can improvise a poem or song about how gorgeous you find them. Linger around the nipples, breasts and sides of the breast, and stroke up under the armpit. Tantalize them with brief contact, moving toward the breasts or nipples and away over the chest and belly. Try feathers, fabrics, fingertips, tongue, hair, or the

bristles on your chin to stroke and caress your lover's breasts. Explore unusual textures to find out what excites them. Alternate between stimulating each breast, or spiral in toward the nipples from the outside.

- Explore the nipples with your tongue, then blow gently on the wet skin. You could have fun licking exotic fruit, such as mango, avocado, or honey from their breasts. Since the breasts are linked to the clitoris and the tip of the penis, a woman can heighten her sensual pleasure by squeezing her love muscle on each in-breath *(see page 162)* and focusing on letting pleasure spread from the heart and breasts down into the genitals.

Tasting nectar: cunnilingus

A prerequisite for giving oral sex is that you perform it with enjoyment, not out of duty. The more you enjoy pleasuring your partners' genitals with your mouth, the greater her pleasure. The more love you impart, the more she will relax into feeling loved.

239

- Allow yourself to really savour her genitals' particular flavour and texture as you lick her from the vagina to the clitoris in long strokes. Breathe out your cool breath on her wet vulval lips, and inhale her unique scent.
- Circle her pearl (clitoris) with your firm tongue, before softly biting or sucking it to encourage her to release her love juices.
- As you taste her love juices, imagine that they are the nectar of bliss. Absorb her vaginal juices and let them nourish you.
- Stay with the style of stimulation that she enjoys, maintaining a steady rhythm as long as you can manage – take over with your fingers if your tongue needs a rest.

Tasting penis: fellatio

In order to inspire your partner, put on some slow, sexy music. Tantalize your lover with a slow and sensuous striptease, revealing your body bit by bit. Then put on a favourite piece of music and dance for her, moving your body freely and allowing your genitals to join the dance. Show off so that your lover can appreciate your body in all its supple inventiveness. Let her witness your celebration of your own erotic being. You also want to arouse her admiration for your member so that she is tempted to take it in her mouth.

The art of oral sex is imbibing your lover's sexual essence as they release their sexual juices. It is an act to be relished. Treat your partner's penis with reverence and love to make him feel great as you handle what to him is his most precious possession.

- Hold his penis and scrotum in the cup of your hands, enjoying getting your hands on all his sex organs at once. Blow through your fingers as he starts to come alive. Gently squeeze and stretch as he swells.
- Play with him, rolling, pressing, stroking or tickling his penis before beginning to caress it with your lips.
- Kiss your lover's penis as if it were his lips. Play your tongue over all its surfaces. Discover the areas your

partner finds particularly sensitive. Press with your mouth and tongue, and suck and lick the tip as if it were an ice-cream cone. Tantalize your partner with swallowing his penis as far as feels comfortable.

- Hold the head of his penis with your fingers while mouthing the sides of the stalk. Lick the underside of his penis, from the seam in his scrotum to the sensitive 'v' shape where the foreskin meets the head of the penis.

- Taste his pre-ejaculate as it oozes from the urethra. If he ejaculates, taste his semen, absorbing its essence into your being. It's up to you if you want to taste a smidgeon or a whole mouthful. It is particularly potent if you accept the semen as his sexual essence. As you swallow, visualize it as nourishing your energy, passion and vitality.

Sexual massage for women

For a woman, it is important to spend time massaging the rest of her body before homing in on her genitals.

Massage her back first so that she closes her eyes and fully relaxes into her own bodily sensations. This will orient her towards receiving. Put all your attention in the palms of your hands and fingertips. After twenty minutes or so, you can start to explore your partner's vagina and vulva, devoting all your attention to what does or doesn't turn her on. Try not to let your mind wander while you are massaging, as this will dilute the enjoyment for your partner. You may want to play relaxing music to help stop you both getting lost in your thoughts.

It's important to discover what she enjoys and what she doesn't like. Keep the channels of communication open, giving each other feedback during and afterwards.

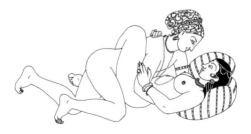

- Make her comfortable, lying with open legs on a nest of quilts and pillows. Sit between her legs and gaze into her eyes, transmitting your love. Rest your left hand over her heart while your right hand cups her pubic mound, reminding her to connect her heart and sexuality.
- After several minutes, massage her whole body gently with massage oil. Play with different strokes and pressures.
- Massage all around the pelvis, and the tops of her thighs. Finish by gently teasing the pubic hair. When your partner asks you to, start massaging her genitals. Pour a small quantity of unscented oil or lubricant into your cupped palm, and anoint the outer lips of the vulva. As you slowly massage the vulva, check that she is enjoying the pace and pressure of your touch. Keep every movement gentle and loving.
- Try different styles of touching, such as delicately pressing each of the outer lips between your thumb and forefinger. Tantalize her by brushing the flesh. Slide your fingers up and down along the lips of the vulva.

- Gently stroke the clitoris in small circles and gentle squeezes. Your partner can tell you what is and what isn't pleasurable. She needs to become absorbed in her sensations rather than staying alert to guide you. Sighs and moans are just as good forms of feedback as a precise commentary – as long as you comprehend the code. Increase her excitement with blended stimulation, using your free hand to stroke and circle a nipple at the same time as her pearl.

- When your partner indicates that she is ready, slowly push your middle finger inside, gently circling the inside of the vagina to discover which areas are pleasurable. The palm of your hand can massage her pubic mound. Vary the depth, speed and pressure of your fingers until you discover what feels good. Try moving your middle finger in a beckoning gesture, rubbing upwards inside her vagina, until you find her exquisitely sensitive areas, such as the g-spot. Spend some time learning how to maintain her arousal as you pleasure this spot *(see page 252)*. Time spent now will repay you in the future.

- Keep breathing and looking into each other's eyes,

massaging until she tells you to stop. Very slowly and gently, remove your finger. Allow her to lie still in your arms and appreciate the afterglow.

Penis massage

As a man, celebrate your penis as a source of enormous pleasure. During the massage, allow yourself to relax into that pleasure. Enjoy erotic stimulation without trying to control it, or hurry on toward sexual release. Be open to appreciating new sensations and moods.

This massage will expand the range of your sexual arousal by exploring the different sensations and moods of your penis during sensual stimulation. Enjoy the sensations without feeling that you have to respond in any way. In advanced Tantric techniques, it is essential that you learn to do nothing. You need to be able to let go of the imperative to perform well.

The goal of penis massage is not orgasm – although that may happen. Try to dismiss thoughts about whether you will or will not have an erection or orgasm; just enjoy letting your genitals be handled in novel ways. In order to relax into receiving, don't direct your partner to stimulate you in the ways that you use during masturbation. Let her try out whatever appeals — although feel free to suggest inventive methods of stimulating you, or specific parts of your genitals that you fancy exploring. You may discover completely new ways of being aroused.

- Your partner lies back on a nest of quilts and pillows. Sit by his side, or between his open legs. Gaze into his eyes, sending him your love. Rest your left hand over his heart while your right hand gently cups his penis and balls, in a wordless reminder to him to connect heart and sexuality. Touch his genitals briefly to acknowledge them before applying massage oil over his body. Anoint his body and touch him all over. Then, ask him if he wants you to massage the rest of his body or his genitals.
- Touch his penis in a sensual, rather than sexual, manner. Encourage him to allow the delicious sensations to spread throughout his body.

- Explore new ways of touching him rather than trying to bring him to orgasm. Start with his penis soft so that you can explore playful ways to touch this sensitive area. Lightly squeeze, rub and massage his penis from the base up. Sensitize his genitals and then stroke his body from his groin outwards, encouraging him to spread the erotic sensations from his genitals throughout the rest of his body.

- Keep coming back to his penis, scrotum and anal area during the massage, and then working outwards again. At frequent intervals throughout the massage, you can help him disperse sexual energy by stroking from his pubic area up the abdomen and chest toward his heart. There you can rest your hand over his heart while you gaze at him lovingly.

- Pay attention to his balls. Hold his scrotum gently in your hand, and let him relax into your holding, trusting you. Softly caress the skin or tease his scrotal hairs. Slide your fingers behind his scrotum towards the anus, and massage him there.

- Tease his penis using your breath, feathers, lips,

fingernails, hair and breasts.

- Hold the base of the penis with one hand and massage the sensitive frenum (on the underside, where the foreskin joins the glans) with the other. Stroke, lick or suck this supremely sensitive area.

Making her come

In terms of ease of orgasm, women's sexual experience can be categorized as pre-orgasmic, sporadically orgasmic, orgasmic, multi-orgasmic and extended pleasure. Before you can go on to the delights of whole-body orgasm and extended sexual pleasure, you need to know how to reliably make your lover come. That means she is at least halfway along this scale of being able to reach her orgasmic potential. If you've never seen her come, you need to start by witnessing her self-pleasuring (as described on page 59).

Unless a woman is blessed with the ability to orgasm easily, most women require at least half an hour of genital stimulation before they can reach a climax. They also need a lot of direct clitoral stimulation, which you can provide with your fingers. This exercise suggests basic techniques to help your woman to her orgasm. Once you've mastered them, you no longer need to concentrate on 'how-to' or count a rhythm of stimulation, or think about the direction in which your breath is moving once you add advanced Tantric techniques like sexual breathing. You will be able to pick and choose from among the exercises on offer in this book, and respond intuitively.

- Relax your lover's whole body with stroking and massage, before sitting on one side so that you can stimulate her pearl (clitoris) with one hand and her vulva with the other.
- Lightly caress her pubic hair, teasing her thighs and the lips of her genitals, using your breath, tongue or fingers to give sensual pleasure.
- After a quarter or half an hour, apply lubricant over her genitals. Circle around her pearl for several minutes, and stroke the top of her clitoris, finding out

what she most enjoys. Don't forget to look at her as you are pleasuring her.

- Try stimulating the top of her pearl with your thumb, while your fingers stroke downward along either side. Keep your stroke slow and steady.

- When your partner is very wet, slowly slide your middle finger into her vagina. It's best to ask if she's ready beforehand – she may want you to spend even more time on pleasuring her clitoris. Gently explore the inside of the vagina in every direction, and slowly massage it. Vary the depth, speed and pressure of your finger. Try small circles, or stroking forwards and backwards with just the tip of your fingers, rather than using an in-out gesture.

- Move your finger around the upper side of her vagina (under the pubic area) with your finger, until you discover the area that she finds most pleasurable. Again, vary the pressure, speed and pattern of movement to pleasure her g-spot. It feels like a slightly rougher, spongy area of tissue the size of a walnut.

- Experiment with all sorts of different strokes, changing

them gradually rather than rapidly, so that your partner has time to relax into the sensations. When your partner tells you that she is really enjoying what you're doing, stay with the same movements for several minutes. If her arousal diminishes, make your movements gentler until she gets excited again, and then return to what worked.

• You can try alternating more pleasurable strokes with lighter versions of the same touch for two or three strokes before returning to the pleasurable pressure. If she does orgasm, continue to rhythmically stroke the g-spot, but lighten your touch. She can build her own arousal by concentrating on breathing in through her vulva, squeezing her love muscle (pelvic floor muscles – *see page 162*) to increase her sensations.

G-spotting

The g-spot – known as the goddess spot or inner pearl – provides sensations as pleasurable as those of the outer

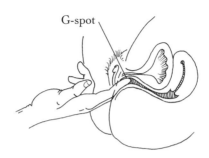

G-spot

pearl (clitoris). Stimulating the g-spot brings women to peak states of arousal. For women who have difficulty achieving orgasm, rubbing the g-spot as well as the clitoris exponentially increases genital pleasure. For women who orgasm easily, you can massage the g-spot to encourage ejaculation *(see female ejaculation, page 256)*. The secret of this exercise is to give your lover more time for genital pleasure than she's ever had before, using your hands and mouth.

• Start with a loving hug and verbally tantalize her by describing what you are planning to do to her.

- Touch her body with love and care, caressing, stroking and massaging her all over. Really concentrate on touching her as slowly, lovingly and sensitively as possible in order to build up sensation and enliven her energy-body. Slow, delicate touch heightens arousal. Pay attention to her whole body, instead of rushing for her sexual organs.

- Anoint her clitoris with an unscented, good-quality massage oil *(see Sexual massage, page 242)*, or perhaps yoghurt if you intend to indulge in oral sex. Spend fifteen or twenty minutes pleasuring her clitoris and external genitals, while you caress her breasts with the other hand, and spend time kissing.

- One of the best ways to give quality clitoral stimulation is with your tongue. For most women the clitoris is the primary means of climaxing – and it's even better with g-spot stimulation at the same time. You should only start massaging this sensitive area once she is feeling very excited and happy to have your finger inside her vagina. Try oral sex with your fingers rubbing her inner pearl at the same time, or rubbing both her clitoris and inner pearl.

- It's best if you know how to find her inner pearl or g-spot from a session of sexual massage, where you explore her sexual anatomy and discover how to turn her on *(see page 242)*. With your finger inside her vagina, explore the spongy tissue of the g-spot, stroking the area in a rhythmic way as her pleasure increases. Try a one-stroke-per-second rhythm to begin with. The combination of rubbing her pearl (clitoris) with a finger inside her vagina to pleasure her g-spot is a marvellous way to encourage an orgasm. For women who orgasm with a combination of clitoral and g-spot stimulation, try pleasuring her manually when she's lying on her front. She can prop her pelvis up on a pillow for better access. With your fingers inside they will naturally press downwards on her g-spot area, while you can rub her clitoris with your thumb. Don't forget to use plenty of lubrication.

- For women who don't enjoy oral sex, try stimulating other areas – lips, nipples, anus …

- When she does start to orgasm, make your touch gentler for up to a minute, but don't stop yet. Maintain a rhythmic pattern of stimulating her that will help prolong her orgasm. Increase the pace and pressure of genital stroking if she asks you to do so. With g-spot arousal her orgasm will be more intense, with exquisite sensations spreading throughout her body.

Female ejaculation

Ejaculate comes from g-spot arousal when the woman is exquisitely turned on. The watery fluid is emitted during orgasm when the g-spot inside the vagina *(see page 252)* has been intensely stimulated for some time. Women who have experienced female ejaculation say that emitting sexual fluids (called nectar, in Tantra) is a sign of tremendous enjoyment. It occurs during sessions of complete abandonment to erotic pleasure, often catching the woman by surprise with the intensity of her response. You can't make it happen, but you can

try and create the right conditions for it to spontaneously occur.

- Get sensual – spend plenty of time on clitoral and g-
  spot stimulation and keep the erotic energy dancing
  between you.
- The woman needs to breathe deeply and let go,
  surrendering herself to pleasure. She imagines herself
  dropping deeper and deeper into her sexual passion.
- She mobilizes her pelvis, rocking and squeezing the
  pelvic floor muscles as she feels her sexual pleasure
  mounting. She vocalizes her excitement. She needs to
  go for whatever really turns her on, without inhibitions. Go with her.
- If she can't sustain the level of arousal, stop trying to
  pleasure her and both sink into the sexual energy you
  have already generated. Look into each other's eyes,
  enjoying the appearance of the sexy, alive creature
  before you. Occasionally rotate your hips, both of you
  breathing down into your genitals and back up
  through the mouth, letting all that lust activate all the

cells in your body. Let your breath mingle as well as your saliva as you kiss. Then start to make love again, with passion and abandon.

Perineum pleasure: making him come

Just because ninety-nine per cent of men like the head of the penis rubbed, don't assume that you know how he comes. The challenge is to explore different ways of pleasuring him. You may discover a way to make him come that he hasn't yet discovered himself. This exercise uses blended stimulation, pleasuring the perineum or inside his anus at the same time as his penis.

- Explore his perineum. Lightly stroke down the shaft of his penis following the base between the testicles, to where his penis starts to swell just in front of his anus. This area feels very enjoyable and often responds to quite deep massage with your fingers or thumb.

Experiment with pressing there in deep, rhythmic strokes, finding a pattern that your partner enjoys and maintaining it.

- Try switching back to the shaft of his penis and ask him what the difference is when pleasuring these two areas. Stimulating the perineum usually reduces the drive to ejaculate, and firm pressure can actually help hold it back. Swap between his penis and perineum to give him mounting waves of pleasure, pulling back before encouraging his arousal to climb again.

Prostate pleasure

The prostate is an often-neglected part of male genitalia. A little walnut-sized gland nestled around the urethra, it produces part of the seminal fluid and, like the penis, contracts during orgasm. Stimulating it during sexual arousal makes orgasm more deep and intense, and prolongs it. The prostate corresponds to the g-spot in women *(see page 252)* – they come from the same tissue.

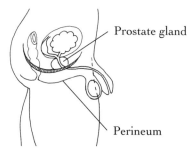

Prostate gland

Perineum

Simultaneously stroking the penis and the prostate area is intensely arousing. You find it by pressing deeply into the perineum (midway between the testicles and anus) or pressing it from inside the anus, if your partner enjoys that. Your partner relaxes his anus while focusing on pleasurable feelings around the prostate area, rather than his penis.

- Sit between his legs for easy access, while he leans back on some cushions.
- Lubricate his pelvic area and genitals with a good oil or other lubricant and play with his scrotum and

perineum (the area behind his testicles, toward his anus), as well as his penis.

- Steady pressure here feels good, or a firm stroking in rhythm with the strokes you're giving his penis. You can press your thumb into the sacred spot while hooking your finger around his penis.

- To build up arousal, you can build up the speed of your rhythmic strokes and then slow down again. He can squeeze his love muscle (pelvic floor muscles – *see page 162)*, and use slow, deep breathing to calm his erotic energy.

- If you don't want him to ejaculate, stop touching his penis and gently pull or stretch the testicles. You can stroke the energy away from the pelvis, especially down his legs and up to his heart area.

- If your partner is really excited, and wants you to stimulate him inside his anus, you can use a latex glove (available from a pharmacy). Lubricate the perineum and anus with massage oil, then ask him to breathe in as you push the tip of your finger inside. Hold your finger just inside the anus until the muscles relax.

When he is relaxed, push your finger in a little more, and gently explore the inside of the anal muscles.

- While his anus is being explored, your partner relaxes into the sensations. If he is at all uncomfortable he should ask you to hold your finger completely still, rather than withdrawing. When he finds the sensations pleasurable again, he can pant to increase his arousal, and squeeze his love muscles around your finger.

Prolonged pleasure and multiple orgasm

All of us would like to make love in a state of high arousal for long periods of time. Learn to delay your orgasm so you both maintain an erotic high, first concentrating on enabling the woman to lengthen her orgasmic response and then prolonging sexual pleasure for both of you. This is a prerequisite for riding the waves of bliss as you both orgasm again and again *(see Riding the wave of bliss, Chapter 7, page 368)*. In these extraordinary lovemaking sessions you can experience whole-body orgasms *(see page 283)*, where your pleasure spreads upwards from your genitals and through the rest of your body.

The next few exercises give tips for men to master the art of ejaculation control.

Delaying ejaculation

For men, ejaculation usually means the rapid decline of sexual excitement. Letting go of the drive to orgasm paradoxically enables you to extend your capacity for erotic pleasure. Learning to delay ejaculation involves developing the capacity to sustain heightened levels of arousal without coming, allowing your lust to ebb and flow.

Sexual arousal comes in waves, with periods when your excitement falls and then climbs again. As you do this exercise and your excitement intensifies, you can focus on breathing through the crest of the wave until your excitement drops, without reaching orgasm. Try to back off if you feel yourself coming to the edge of an orgasm, and focus instead on relaxing into your arousal.

Slow down your breathing rather than speeding up. Keep your movements very slow, and breathe slowly and deeply in order to avert the approach of orgasm.

- Caress your partner's genitals for some time. Lightly brush the pubic area, playing with light, teasing strokes.
- Once your partner is aroused and wanting genital stimulation, touch the rest of his body instead of giving him sexual release straight away.
- Again, tease his sexual organs with the lightest of touch (or blow), before anointing his penis, scrotum and anus with lubricant.
- Stroke his penis along the seam from the glans along the scrotum, all the way to his anus. This part, the root of the penis, often doesn't get enough attention. Alternate between stimulating his genitals and stroking his excitement away from his chest and upper body or down the legs.
- Stimulate him right up to the verge of orgasm several times, stopping each time he feels he might ejaculate. Stop, without bringing him to orgasm.

Delay tactics through self-pleasuring

When you learn to delay orgasm, you can hold on to pleasure, prolonging arousal for you and your partner. While sometimes you may want a quickie sex, delay tactics are most potent in the context of regular and satisfying, lengthy lovemaking. If you find it difficult holding back, needing to use unsexy thoughts or fantasies to keep yourself from coming, you need to practise delay tactics during self-pleasuring sessions.

Try this self-management technique to contain your orgasm.

- Pleasure yourself with your hands, using a good lubricant.
- During self-pleasuring, repeatedly stimulate yourself to the very edge of orgasm, even up to the point that contractions start at the base of your penis.
- Try to keep yourself on the edge for at least half an hour, before allowing yourself to come. Once you can

self-pleasure for half an hour without ejaculating, you should be able to go on as long as you want when making love with your partner.

Deferred gratification

It's very important for the man to know what it is like to make love without having an orgasm, especially if his partner finds it difficult reaching one herself. This exercise is also helpful if you have problems sustaining an erection, or feel anxiety about it.

Tantric sex involves coming together, rather than coming. Try to be together in the experience of sex rather than going for what you want and leaving your partner high and dry. Anyway, there are rewards in it for you. If you can let go of the drive towards your own orgasm you can explore whatever arises spontaneously between you. Giving up your attachment to orgasm paradoxically allows you to get more pleasure from other aspects of your sexuality. You are able to immerse yourself in your whole-body sensations, and use this sexual energy to nourish your loving connection with your mate. You can explore the subtle sensations produced by small movements of your pelvis, your love (pelvic floor) muscles, and altering your breathing.

- Start to make love any way you like. As you feel your excitement climbing, stop moving and lie still with the penis inside the vagina, just experiencing the sensations without having to create more. Use the minimal movement you need just to maintain an erection. Don't worry about losing your erection, as you can re-stimulate it.

- The woman uses blended stimulation when she wants his levels of excitement to climb rapidly, where you rub both the tip of the penis and the perineum together *(see page 258)*. 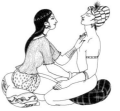 As you massage his external prostate, he can rhythmically squeeze his own love muscle. If he enjoys anal stimulation, you can massage his prostate gland with your finger from inside his anus. You can alternate between pleasuring his prostate, and then pleasuring his penis for maximum pleasure.

- Once he's excited bring his penis inside you again, without much thrusting. See what it feels like allowing your genitals to inter-penetrate and create a bridge for the exchange of energies. Surrender yourselves to the process and let go of your urge to orgasm.

The next few exercises describe techniques to facilitate multiple orgasms in both women and men, and how to direct the energy of your synchronized orgasms into explosive whole-body experiences.

G-spotting during sex

When pleasured, the g-spot produces sexual bliss. It's not a button that will automatically tip you into multiple orgasms, but a period of rhythmic massage will intensify genital pleasure and expand your orgasmic sensations. G-spot stimulation during intercourse vastly increases your pleasure. Stimulation of the g-spot during prolonged pleasuring leads to female ejaculation *(see page 256)*, the liquid Tantrics call divine nectar.

In this exercise, you use blended stimulation for women, simultaneously stroking the clitoris and g-spot by slipping a finger inside her. Women may need direct clitoral stimulation during intercourse rather than relying on the indirect pressure offered during intercourse. She can rub her own clitoris if you don't have a free hand.

- Once your man has located your g-spot with his fingers *(see page 252)*, try to rub the same sensitive area when his penis is inside you. The best position is usually on top, sometimes leaning backward, or even facing backwards. Experiment with lovemaking positions that change the angle of penetration to give you most pleasure.
- While on top, pump your love muscle – contract and release the muscles around your vagina and anus

about twice per second. You can pump your love muscle and rotate your pelvis against your partner's pubic area so that it massages your clitoris.

- For deep penetration, place a pillow under your hips and rest your legs along the front of his chest. Your man can try short deep thrusts, without withdrawing his penis much – this can be very stimulating for you without giving him a quick orgasm. Or, lie with your buttocks raised in the air exposing your vulva, resting your head on your crossed arms.

- Some women prefer penetration to be less deep. Try lying with the woman's back facing your partner for rear entry.

- If you need your partner to maintain intercourse without having an orgasm himself, he should only withdraw his penis minimally between thrusts. If he uses short thrusts with his penis remaining deep inside this will reduce his stimulation while still plea-suring your g-spot area.

Multiple orgasm for women

Enjoying multiple orgasm has a lot to do with good sex techniques, as well as a loving and attentive partner. Orgasm itself can be prolonged in waves of deepening pleasure, called a valley orgasm, where the orgasm keeps going for some minutes.

- Start by caressing, stroking and massaging your lover's body all over. Put all your attention into your fingertips. Concentrate totally on touching her as slowly, lovingly and sensitively as possible in order to build up sensation and enliven her energy-body.
- Stroke her whole body with slow, delicate touch to heighten her arousal.
- When your partner wants you to caress her genitals, rub a good-quality lubricant all round her vulva. Touch her in the way and places that she likes; thighs, pubic mound and anus. Tease the pearl (clitoris) by brushing it and circling around it with one, two or more fingers.

- Experiment with light strokes, maintaining a steady rhythm of once a second as she rolls her pelvis around, moving or arching her back and squeezing her love (pelvic floor) muscle as you pleasure her.
- When she asks you to enter her, slip one or two fingers inside. Stroke her g-spot, which is in the front and upward in the vagina – at the end of your finger-tips. Rub her g-spot by twiddling the end of your finger rather than using an in-and-out motion to mimic intercourse. Alternatively, try sweeping your fingers in a circular gesture. Once you've found out what feels intensely pleasurable and where, continue the rhythmic stimulation you were using on her clitoris. Let the pleasure intensify.
- She can rub her own clitoris at the same time as you are stroking her g-spot inside the vagina, which leaves you with a free hand to caress her breasts or thighs.
- When your partner starts to orgasm, focus your attention on rubbing her g-spot rhythmically with one or two fingers. Hook your fingers upward, rubbing the top wall of her vagina where it feels extremely pleasurable,

to increase the depth of orgasm. As she begins the contractions of her orgasm, rhythmically stroke the g-spot quite firmly. Maintain the same rhythm.

- As you continue stimulating, she may go into deeper pelvic contractions. As they lessen, lighten your stimulation of the g-spot and try to pleasure her clitoris again until you feel her orgasm building again. As you feel her internal contractions, go back to stimulating her g-spot as she continues her orgasm. You can prolong her orgasm and learn how to give her multiple orgasms by alternating between the vagina and clitoris for over a quarter of an hour.

Multiple orgasm for men: orgasm without ejaculation

Sexual pleasure is much more than being able to come as quickly as possible.

If you want to learn how to have multiple orgasms like your partner, you need to learn how to reach a peak of sexual arousal and then plateau again without ejaculating. When you do this repeatedly you can learn to dance on the edge of your orgasm, letting orgasmic contractions start without going on to ejaculate. By lengthening the moment between orgasm and ejaculation, you can extend and deepen your experience of orgasm, experiencing a deeper and more satisfying type of climax, called a valley orgasm.

You can learn to expand the length of your orgasmic contractions from seconds to minutes or even longer, maintaining a high level of arousal without physically ejaculating. In this way, you can enjoy making love more often and for longer. This technique promises literally endless pleasure. Once you have learned how to have orgasms without ejaculation, you'll be able to sustain prolonged intercourse at high levels of arousal for as long as you choose.

- Lie between his legs with your head on one thigh so you will be able to stimulate his penis with one hand and his testicles, scrotum and prostate with the other, as well as being able to lick his penis comfortably.

- Before touching his genitals, spend several moments connecting his sex and heart chakras (energy centres) by holding one hand cupping his balls and penis, with the other lying palm down between his breasts as a reminder to open the heart.

- Start by lubricating his pelvic area and genitals with massage oil, and play with his penis to arouse him. Don't become too genitally focused – keep backing off from intense penile pleasure by drawing his excitement away from his genitals by stroking away. Then touch his scrotum gently and press into his perineum more firmly, which stimulates his prostate from outside. Try steady pressure with your thumb. If he enjoys anal stimulation, gently rub the internal prostate spot – about half a finger-length inside the anus, with your finger crooked up toward you. He can guide you to where it feels especially pleasurable, and tell you what sort of pressure to use.

- When he gets very excited, switch back to his penis, but slowly, so that he doesn't ejaculate. Tantalize him, building up this pleasure and then swapping back to stimulating his prostate. Alternate between his penis and prostate, between areas that are more pleasurable and those that are slightly less pleasurable, to give him waves of pleasure.

- To increase his excitement, just increase the speed of your strokes. He can squeeze his love muscle (pelvic floor muscles), and alternate between rapid and deep breathing. To reduce his excitement, slow the pace and pressure of your strokes while he breathes deeply.
- To stop him ejaculating, stop stimulating his penis and use your hands to stroke the energy away from his pelvis while he concentrates on not ejaculating. Use slow breathing to slow your contractions right down; squeeze your love muscle and hold to prevent orgasm.
- Together, build up to high levels of arousal, then come down again, before building up and cooling down several more times. The woman can play with keeping him on the verge of an orgasm for at least half an hour, allowing him to repeatedly start orgasmic contractions without ejaculating.

Your partner needs to alert you to when contractions start at the base of his penis, around the prostate and anus. By paying more attention to these contractions he can let them go a little bit further each time before pulling back, until they build in intensity and roll into a repeated orgasm that goes on for some time without ejaculating.

After some practice, he'll be able to maintain high levels of arousal without needing to ejaculate, and experience a series of orgasms similar to those experienced by multi-orgasmic women.

Going into the valley: prolonging orgasm

The valley orgasm describes a delicious sense of relaxation into erotic pleasure that often occurs naturally in lengthy bouts of lovemaking. In the valley orgasm, you have a number of orgasms without your pleasure dropping between orgasm. Your sexual energy is contained rather than dissipated through ejaculation, so that you can climb to higher and higher peaks of pleasure. Men achieve this by holding back their ejaculation *(see above and pages 263, 273)*; women achieve it by continuing genital stimulation after the first orgasm. After the briefest pause, carry on with either intercourse or stimulation of the inner pearl (g-spot: *see page 252*) or outer pearl (clitoris).

- The man keeps bringing the woman to orgasm while he holds back. The woman surrenders totally to pursuing her own sexual fulfilment, while the man concentrates on facilitating the ebb and flow of her orgasmic process while making sure he doesn't ejaculate.
- She builds her sexual arousal with sexual breathing and love-muscle pumps *(see page 164)* as he pleasures her clitoris and g-spot, first with his fingers and later with his penis. He brings her to orgasm manually and then you both relax together as she comes down from her climax. He leaves his finger inside her vagina as her contractions die away.

- After less than a minute, he starts to stimulate her again, introducing his penis. The aim is to bring her to a peak of arousal, then drop into a short plateau before climbing to ever higher peaks of arousal.
- The orgasmic process can be extended from a few seconds to as much as half an hour. The man contains his impulse to orgasm by firmly clenching the love muscles at the base of his penis and around the anus, holding his breath and rolling his eyes upward. She can help by firmly pressing the perineum (the area between the anus and the testicles) to lock the excitement in.

Synchronized orgasm

Once you have both developed control and flexibility over the orgasmic process, you can work on synchronizing your orgasms so that you both climax together. Most of the couple visualizations that focus on orgasmic breathing and moving energy through your joined bodies require you to be able to reach orgasm simultaneously. This makes the exercises infinitely more potent and ensures you reach a state of bliss together – rather than one of you being spaced out while the other languishes on the shores of their disappointment.

When you understand the pace of your partner's sexual arousal and are familiar with a range of methods for bringing your partner to orgasm, you should be able to determine the moment at which each of you will come. With a little practice you will be able to synchronize your orgasms reliably, leaving you both free to concentrate on the visualizations demonstrated in the following exercises.

A visualization for extended pleasure

Sex is a powerful current of energy flowing through us all. Tantra believes that sexual congress balances and harmonizes energy, and that sexual intercourse can be healing.

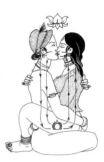

You can experience this by visualizing an exchange of erotic energy during intercourse. Visualization is an essential Tantric technique. It helps you contain and deepen your sensual pleasure rather than hurtling toward orgasmic release. This exercise is very healing when you've experienced sexual problems, or are trying to recover from wounding emotional experiences such as infidelity. You can continue the meditation after you both come, if you choose.

- Start with an open-heart meditation *(see page 187)*. This helps you to celebrate your lovemaking with joy and delight, opening your heart to each other to share your mutual pleasure and increase your receptivity to sexual energy.
- Let your love flow freely as you meditate, and celebrate your desire for each other.
- Encourage the excitement in your penis to spread

outward, enveloping your whole body as an enormous phallus. Imagine that it is radiant with love as you penetrate her; let waves of love pour into her body from your penis as you make love.

- The woman embraces the man's phallus and sends him waves of love through her vagina, with each out-breath. Open your genitals and pelvis to receiving your partner's sexual energy through his penis. As a man, open yourself fully to embracing your partner's loving sexual energy through your penis.

- Open your hearts to each other, and let each other's sexual energy course through your bodies, permeating every cell.

- Relax into the gentle peace and harmony of the experience. Let the fine energy you create through your loving sex stream through you. Feel the love in your partner's genitals as you make love.

- If you don't need to worry about birth control, this is a lovely extension of the visualization. After ejaculating, continue moving to mix the semen together with female ejaculate. Women can use the love-muscle squeeze to milk their partner of his juices *(see page 162)*. Men can squeeze their love muscle and imagine sucking up the love juices, as if their penis were a straw.

Whole-body orgasm

In whole-body orgasm, the exquisite sensations around your genitals spread up and through the rest of your body in waves of energy called streamings, even without orgasm. Orgasm and ejaculation are just natural extensions of these. In Tantra you can send the sexual energy up the conduit from the base of the spine to the crown of the head, flushing your whole body with waves of orgasmic pleasure. You need to synchronize your levels of arousal at this stage of your lovemaking so that you can move into orgasm together. The best position to facilitate waves of sexual energy washing upwards is to sit in the sexual posture described on page 76 (half lotus) or yab-yom *(page 167)*.

Learning to prolong your pleasure means you can

increase your sensitivity and abandon yourself to waves of intense pleasure. Without panting and jerking in preparation for climax, the man melts into a state of relaxed arousal, choosing whether or not to orgasm. Your penis becomes supremely sensitive: a single drop of lubricant, a light blowing breath, or the slightest touch of a tongue gives intense pleasure. For the woman, her sexual excitement can keep climbing, and she can luxuriate in her sensual reverie while her partner also lies with her, concentrating on his subtle sensations. Let the sensations in your genitals spread deliciously through your body.

- Bring yourselves to the edge of orgasm, and then stop. Lie there for a while, feeling the heightened energy spreading throughout your body.
- Concentrate on not ejaculating – not by thinking about something non-sexual, but by imagining your sexual excitement moving away from your penis. Imagine heat or light spreading upwards, into the area of your heart. Slow your breathing to slow your heart

rate right down. Imagine your sexual pleasure spreading from your penis throughout your whole body. Imagine it spreading up into you heart as your pleasure climbs.

- If you feel you are nearing orgasm, the man should stop and squeeze the love (pelvic floor) muscle and hold it firmly. Both of you imagine that your excitement is a stream of heat. Breathe more slowly and deeply. With every in-breath, imagine that you are pulling the heat up from your heart towards your forehead. Let the stream of energy drop back down to your genitals with your exhalation. Send the out-breath back to your forehead, passing through your hearts. This encourages your erotic fervour to expand upwards.

- When you do orgasm, imagine that your orgasm is pouring out of the crown of your head. If you have been having a prolonged lovemaking session both of you should be having a long orgasm or a series of orgasms in which you can both be meditating together.

Circular-breathing orgasm

As you make love, focus on the way energy is circulated within you as one body when you exchange breaths. In this exercise you join your physical and energy-bodies in a complete embrace, which sets up an energy circuit between your joined genitals and mouths. This intensifies pre-orgasmic pleasure, deepening and prolonging orgasm deliciously.

• Join your mouths together, circulating your breathing: as your partner exhales, breathe in their warm breath,

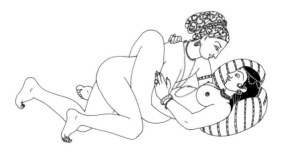

and send it down to your genitals. As you breathe out, push the sexual energy out through your tilted pelvis onto your partner's genitals. From there your partner will draw the energy up to their mouth. Cover your partner's lips with your own, completely sealing the breath. The man inhales through his mouth as the woman exhales through hers. Then the man exhales as the woman inhales through her mouth.

- Now close your eyes and continue the circular breathing for up to ten to fifteen minutes, creating a heady state of excitement. Occasionally inhale through your nostrils to bring in some fresh air. With your mouths together, you become one body, circulating breath between your genitals and the area of your throat and mouth. Touch the tip of your partner's tongue with your own.

- If the woman is less excited than the man, stop moving at frequent intervals during lovemaking to let your erotic sensations spread through your body. This allows the man's penile excitement to subside a bit before you start to move again.

- When you're both feeling near orgasm, close your eyes, roll your eyeballs upwards and squeeze your love (pelvic floor) muscles to contain your sexual excitement as you hold your breath. (One of you will be holding your breath in, the other will be holding without any air in their lungs. When it's no longer comfortable, take a breath, and your partner will exhale, and hold.) Relax the rest of your body, and just allow the energy to stream upwards through you.

- Remain quite still for several minutes, breathing naturally through your nostrils.

- When your excitement has faded, build up your erotic excitement again by moving your bodies. Again, join your lips to seal this energy in your united bodies, one partner inhaling as the other exhales. Now you can circulate the energy right up to the crown of your head, imagining that your whole energy system is one circulating ball of bliss. Relax into the blissful feelings of being at one with the world.

Exploding orgasm

In this exercise, I have concentrated on the male experience, but it assumes that both of you are reaching orgasm together. Exploding orgasm is Tantra-speak for sending the energy of your orgasms upward through the crown of your head when you climax, rather than downwards and through your genitals. First you generate a pool of sensual pleasure, fed by your erotic excitement. You contain it within your bodies, letting passion mount until it fills your being, embracing your lover as you both move toward sexual completion. Through breath control you draw the blissful sensations upwards from the genitals into your heart, and eventually up to the crown of your head. Both of you imagine this movement of energy as you have a synchronized orgasm. Let the orgasmic energy at the crown of your heads merge and pool.

• Build up sexual arousal through stroking your lover's penis, scrotum and perineum. Use the technique of blended stimulation – stimulating both together, or alternating between one and the other. The idea is to keep him in a high state of pleasure for as long as possible without letting him slip into orgasm. That means backing off from stimulating his penis when he gets overexcited. Some men say that pressing into the perineum (over the area of the prostate) stops them coming because it quickly switches attention away from the penis. You can also use your hands to stroke the energy over his skin and away from his pelvis.

- You can try to stop orgasm by bearing down on your love muscles as if you are straining to push out a bowel movement. Then completely relax those same muscles, and focus on dispersing your excitement upwards through your body.

- During your orgasmic contractions, imagine your orgasm rushing up from your genitals up to the crown of your head. Feel the energy pulsations in your head as you come. Doing this draws the blissful sensations upwards from your genitals into your heart, and eventually up to the crown of your head.

Quickie sex

This might seem like a contradiction in terms, as Tantric sex requires attention to the subtle movements of desire and pleasure in your body. However, if you are having regular lengthy lovemaking sessions you can use quickies to dip into the strong current of sexual energy underpinning your life and use it to enhance the rest of your day. If you're used to taking plenty of time and being subtle and refined in your attention to each other's needs, your sexual energy can be tapped quickly – and it may only take a few moments to reach high levels of arousal.

You may not have time for a longer lovemaking session, but quickie sex can sexualize your whole day. Through touching base with your sexuality you connect with your core self, stoking up your sexual fire and reminding yourself of your innate energy. If the sex you have is enlivening you, it doesn't matter if it's over quickly; however, if you feel depleted or shut down by sexual or emotional disappointment, you should avoid quickies.

Even when sex is fast, it's still important to really connect with your lover, to open your hearts in acknowledgement of the importance of sexuality in your life and relationship. In my opinion, quick fucks only work if you are having lots of regular sex; unless a woman orgasms easily it's more difficult to satisfy her during quick sex, and she'll become resentful and withdrawn if sex isn't fulfilling.

Afterplay

Just as sex starts long before you take your clothes off, afterplay continues long after your orgasm dies away. Orgasm is used as a gateway to bliss – so you'll miss out on a great deal if you just roll over and go to sleep. This is a special time for deepening your intimacy and joining your energy-body with that of your mate. Post-orgasm is a perfect time for meditation, when you can enter some rarefied states of consciousness. You can simply use one of the connecting exercises in Step 2 *(see pages 66, 78)* or the Light laundry in Step 1 *(see page 16)*.

Re-stimulate a whole-body orgasm

Your mind is the key to the best sex in your life. You have the capacity to give yourself an orgasm through the power of your mind. Some people can have an orgasm while being pleasured, some from just thinking about their pleasure. This exercise uses a combination of sexual breathing techniques together with visualization techniques and pelvic floor squeezes to create a whole-body orgasm.

You can use your sexual process to reach blissful ecstasy without making love. If you need a head start and have developed multi-orgasmic capacity, try and have an energy orgasm following the first genital one. Use the delightful sensations and awareness of the movement of sexual energy through your body to fuel an energy orgasm, without requiring any further physical stimulation.

• Don't withdraw after intercourse. Remain seated with your genitals connected. If you are doing this exercise without your genitals joined, it helps if you are seated wrapped around each other, in a half lotus, rebuilding your arousal together. A double energy-body is doubly powerful.

- Generate sexual energy by breathing deeply into your genitals. As you do so, imagine them getting hotter.

- Try to breathe rapidly, imagining the energy snaking up from your genitals. Rhythmically squeeze the love muscles of your pelvic floor to help the excitement climb.

- Let your breathing rate calm down again, then join your mouths and tongues together and circulate your breath between you as described on page 286. Keep your mouths together. Imagine an oval tube linking you, with energy circulating as you breathe in turns.

- If you squeeze your pelvic floor muscles when you are in a heightened state of sexual arousal, you may be able to reactivate the fine contractions that herald orgasm. Concentrate on pulling the pleasure upwards from your genitals as the orgasmic process unfolds. Let your sexual energies blend and merge above your head. Nourish your unified being with this fine sexual energy.

Tantric sex

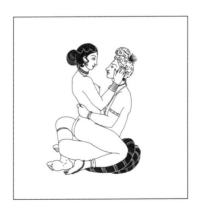

Bringing the sacred into your relationship

The final step in materializing bliss is to integrate what you have absorbed from this book. The first Step explained how to love yourself well in order to love your partner in a consistently caring way. Remember that the source of your capacity for love lies in your own deeper nature. This essence is revealed in periods of contemplation or meditation.

Step 2 revealed the importance of making an authentic connection with your beloved; in Steps 3 and 4 you explored sensation and your desire for each other. In Step 5, you learned to dissolve emotional blocks to sexual fulfilment, and in Step 6, the sexual techniques that keep you orgasmically close.

In this Step, you bring divine bliss into your relationship. Discover joy, and find a wellspring of devotion within you. In the Rosebud meditation *(see page 97)* you channelled all your petty complaints and sense of irritation into loving kindness – this is an aspect of your devotional side. The capacity for devotion is considered a sign of soul awakening, along with the qualities of altruism and compassion *(see A meditation for compassion, page 213)*. This is the reason why the most profound exercises in this book are those where you imagine yourself, your partner and then both of you together as divinities – see *Imagine yourself as a divinity (page 323)*. These exercises offer a simple technique for radically transforming your relationship into a chalice, or container, for bliss.

Tantric masters promise that when you are spiritually awakened, states of joy and bliss spontaneously arise. But you can activate these experiences yourself rather than passively waiting for them to occur. Meditation is the path to awakening your consciousness, allowing you to access bliss. This book has presented a range of meditations, including breath work and visualizations, to give you a taste of the bliss that Tantric masters describe as your birthright. You don't need to believe in bliss in order for these exercises to work – but be warned that using Tantra is likely to produce a spiritual perspective on your life.

Integrating sex

Soulful sex puts you on the fast track to improving your relationship and deepens intimacy. When you open emotionally during sex, your sexual passion is available to nourish your heart. It encourages you to open to the delight that is yours to experience with your lover. You can integrate the bliss that you uncover during lovemaking into the rest of your day.

Sexual love leaves you receptive to the personal love of your partner and more aware of the transpersonal nature of love. Through sex, you can open to the experience of love as your fundamental reality. Such glimpses are so seductive that they inspire you to weave your relationship into a vibrant, organically growing fabric. Your relationship evolves into a flexible, nurturing, passionate and compassionate expression of who you are.

Integrating love

To welcome Tantra into your relationship is to make a heartfelt commitment to a radically different way of being together – a way of relating that is full of pleasure and possibility.

It is easy to simplify love and loving others. Make time for the basic essentials in life – your family and friends, sharing meals, creating a loving home, spending time sharing and caring. Tantra brings you an awareness that you are intimately interconnected to a network of other people. You are not an isolated individual, locked up in your own private world; integrate this awareness into your thinking.

Consider how to generate more love in your relationship so that it touches those around you, allowing them to participate in its positive, healing energy. Love is not just about your romantic relationship; you can create a Tantric attitude toward everyone in your circle. Your love needs to radiate: this means remaining open to other people and being available to meet their needs.

Think about how you can be of service to your community, whether your community consists of friends, extended family or a wider social group.

- Try to shift your self-centred perspective to an altruistic sense of purpose. Prioritize your positive feelings towards others, connecting your love with your wider community.
- Suspend your judgment of others, and accept them as they are.
- Try to engage with people at the level of their needs and concerns. Behave in an open-hearted, warm and generous way; cultivate kindness, caring and consideration in your interactions. Encourage others through your warmth and loving acceptance.
- Being supportive means providing others with the opportunity to be themselves, rather than trying to fix their problems.

You can develop all these attitudes by bringing them into your partnership. When you decide to use your relationship as a central tool for learning and growth, you may find that any neglected aspects of your partnership resurface. For example, the ability to be yourself with your lover may become a crucial issue *(see Making an authentic connection, Step 2, page 66)*.

You can use this book to help you focus on any areas of your life and relationship that need attention – many of the healing exercises in Step 5 *(see pages 184, 189, 190, 198 for example)* are designed for this purpose.

In all spiritual traditions, love implies egolessness – letting go of your notion of yourself as a separate individual. In letting go of your concern with how other people see you, you are less likely to be alienated from your own authentic nature by conforming to social pressures, or by your own ideas about your identity or what you or your partner should be. According to all spiritual traditions, your own authentic nature is love. In love, you don't feel separated from your partner or from anyone else.

Integrating love involves healing your experience of separation from your divine self as well as from your self and your lover. Your body needs to be reunited with the mind, your heart with your soul, the divine with your daily life, and the female with the male.

There is a similarity between longing for a partner and a sense of spiritual longing (for a sense of purpose, meaning, or a direct experience of the divine presence). If you are stuck in longing for a better relationship, try to direct this longing towards exploring your creativity and the creative energy of the cosmos. Use your longing to deepen your soul's journey. In concentrating on centring yourself, you focus your sense of longing on deepening your contact with your soul.

Affirmations

Contemplate the following in your meditative practice.

Through meditation, I become quieter in my life.

I accept the way things are in my life.

I no longer see things in terms of opposites; I accept the non-duality of masculine and feminine principles.

In our relationship, we accept the emotional states that arise between us.

What is consciousness?

Consciousness is another term to describe the energy field that makes up existence. Each of us is a local manifestation of this energy field. That implies that we are fundamentally inseparable from everything else on this planet. Opening the chakra, or energy centre, located at the crown of your head means opening up to universal energy so that you feel a part of the vast network that supports life.

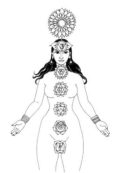

Opening your consciousness to the experience of bliss is what

303

sexual practices are all about in Tantra. Bliss is not just what you experience in the briefest moment of orgasm, but a more pervasive pleasure which tinges your being ruby red *(see the Heart drops exercise on page 366)*.

Consciousness is a lived experience rather than a mental quality. Through consciousness, you find the answers about the nature of existence inside yourself rather than outside. Simply being allows the wisdom of your inner nature to emerge into conscious awareness. This is why it is important to cultivate doing nothing (just being) rather than constantly being busy doing activities in life. In order to become wise, allow your inner wisdom to guide you.

Enlightened humans say that when you are in harmony with the underlying nature of reality (which is bliss) you experience it as an integration of being, consciousness and pure joy.

Enlightenment isn't an unobtainable transformation of awareness. It is simply settling into a receptive openness – where you are open to everything that is happening around you. Those who've been there talk about it as a waking up to the blindingly obvious. Life isn't radically different, but your experience of it is.

Enlightenment can also be described as your full presence to yourself, your unbroken awareness of the fullness of your being, in which your compassion can flow forth freely in accordance with your abilities and your purpose in life. However, this doesn't necessarily mean that you are unruffled by painful experience.

Only mistaken ideas about your identity and purpose in life stand in the way of your divine nature shining through. Rigid and defensive patterns of relating can be cleared though meditation practice. Otherwise, your deepest nature may produce all sorts of turbulence in its uncompromising attempts to find expression. Breakups, breakdowns and mid-life crises are some of the usual ways that the stirrings of your deepest self impacts on your carefully controlled world. These can be potent states of opening, in spite of the fact that you may feel that you are falling to pieces as your familiar world disintegrates into something that is chaotic, but also more intense.

Non-doing

In order to have an amazingly different experience of sexual energy, try to make love with an attitude of non-doing.

Non-doing means letting go of the desire for excitement or the goal of orgasm. There is an art to doing nothing more than connecting and waiting to see what develops. Neither of you taking the lead. Letting feelings arise and flower before you act on them.

Make love without any sense of doing, and without a need to orgasm. Start to make love, and then just stop and lie still with genitals still connected, simply experiencing the sensations without having to pursue more pleasure.

- You lie (or sit) with your partner, just feeling their presence, and connecting sexually.
- Simple touch on your skin can be extremely erotic.
- Prolong your pleasure by taking time.
- Take breaks, deferring ecstasy.
- Squeeze your pelvic floor muscles *(see page 162)* to improve arousal and pleasure.

- Let go of performance imperative. Let go of the idea of doing, and just try to be. In lovemaking, this requires paying attention to what is happening between you right now, allowing yourselves to explore whatever arises. Become absorbed in the sensations, textures, qualities and feelings generated by your lovemaking. Keep stopping during touching or intercourse and sense the energy created between you. Simply enjoy the sensations and emotional connection.

- When you start to move again, explore the subtle sensations produced by minimal adjustments of the position of your pelvis, and your pelvic floor or love muscles. Move your love muscle rather than your pelvis to stimulate sexual arousal. If you want to arouse your sexual fire, use pelvic pumps *(see page 164)*. Don't worry about losing your erection – the woman can guide the penis into her vagina when soft *(see page 224)*.

- Maintain eye contact. Stay totally relaxed – it's important not to tense your muscles as you usually do, striving toward an orgasm.

- Keep taking breaks, letting your erotic pleasure suffuse you. You will find that your erotic pleasure gets more intense each time you start to touch each other again.
- While your genitals are connected, concentrate on the energy exchange between you. Stay focused on the breathing, rather than rushing for an orgasm. Take your time. You may want to move into a sitting position with your legs wrapped around each other. Visualize your breath swinging down all the energy centres in your body as you breathe out, and up through those of your partner – in a u-shape linked by your sex.
- During periods of intercourse stop, slowly building your arousal and resting in it. If you are on the verge of an orgasm try to remain in this state of arousal. As soon as one or two contractions happen, relax your abdominal muscles and breathe slowly. Try to spend at least half an hour playing on the verge of your pleasure. You may also rest and begin again later if you like.
- Instead of going after a climax, the orgasm happens itself and your body responds by melting into it.

Circle of breath

- Start by gazing at each other.
- Focus on listening to each other's breath. Let your focused attention screen out any background noise. Make your breath one breath. As your breath slows, his follows, keeping pace.
- Breathing in this way is so gently intimate that it is like witnessing the essence of each other. There is no need to do anything else. Just look. Just breathe. Breathe into your heart area, directing your breath to fill your heart with loving energy.
- Bring your mouths together, joining lips. After several minutes, inhale your partner's exhaled air, renewing it and returning it to them. Continue for half an hour, offering each other your breath as if it were the elixir of life.
- Through this breathing, where you inhale each other, focus on incorporating each other into your cells. Enjoy the heady sensation induced through the reduction in oxygen levels. Take a breath of fresh air

through the side of your joined lips every so often, without breaking the connection of your two lips.

Variation

This breathing exercise is also wonderful during intercourse, with the woman on the man's lap *(see Circular breathing during lovemaking, Step 6, page 286)*. Use the circle of breath to build your sexual arousal rather than relying on genital friction.

Love and ecstasy

When you embark upon the Tantric path, you begin a journey that involves uncovering your true nature. It is not about transforming yourself, but revealing what has always been present within. Those who have experienced this tell us that it feels like finding your way back home.

Ecstasy means being able to stand outside yourself, and become more than yourself. You identify with your authentic nature, dropping the false image of yourself imposed upon you by you, by others or social convention.

Sex is a gateway to ecstasy; you can access ecstasy by discovering that bliss is part of your essential nature.

What is bliss?

Fundamentally, bliss is loving connection. Bliss describes a state of deep connection with your partner, and through them, the rest of the world. In sexual bliss, you contact the energy field all around you.

Tantric practices, as you have seen throughout this book, use breath work and visualization to help you attain a state of bliss.

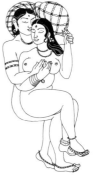

Bliss is an energy-body. Through Tantra, you transform your two physical bodies into a unified energy-body. During post-coital energy meditation, you can see yourselves as a single body of bliss *(see page 345)*. The sexual techniques described in this book culminate in an exercise called Riding the wave of bliss *(see*

page 368). Through this and other bliss exercises, Tantra uses your propensity to reach states of bliss through sex to help you discover at-one-ment.

Bliss is ...

Bliss is making a commitment to love.

Always behaving in a loving way toward your partner.

Holding back on criticism or put-downs.

Returning to loving thoughts inside.

Generating sexual bliss

Breathing and visualization exercises are designed to draw energy upwards and develop a more sensitive, subtle, evolved sexuality.

Open your heart to nourish your loving emotions.
Build your sexual energy by connecting it with love,
enriching your relationship. When you link sex with
heart and spirit, you open your body to the powerful
energy fuelled by your erotic drive. In this ritual, you
power your sexual centre by breathing in and out of
your genitals, then drawing that energy into your heart
to activate your love. You visualize that your love unites
above the crown of your head as you make love.

• Stand facing each other, and gaze into each other's
  eyes. Let loving feelings flower as you connect with
  your partner.
• Inhale together, while you imagine the breath entering
  through your genitals. Visualize that you are breathing
  in through your vagina or – for men – your perineum,
  (between the anus and scrotum) and pulling the breath
  up through the centre of your body, coming to rest in
  the area of your heart by the end of each inhalation.
• Pause at the end of the in-breath, letting your sexually
  charged breath fill your heart.

- Release your breath to drop down through the centre of your body towards the tailbone and out through your genitals.
- Once you both feel your heart is warm and loving, move your right hand to your partner's chest, laying it over their heart. With your next out-breath, visualize the energy streaming from your heart into their heart. With your in-breath, inhale the heart energy that is streaming from your partner, and send it back down to your genitals.
- As you continue breathing in this way for several minutes, focus on letting sexual energy build in your pelvis. With each inhalation, draw this erotic energy up to your heart with each breath. Remain in eye contact with your partner, sharing your joint desire to unite your sexuality and spirituality.
- Come into sexual union, with the woman sitting on her partner's lap, his penis inside.
- Imagine the energy rising to the crown of your head as you make love.
- You should be able to feel energy streaming up from

your pelvis, as the sexual charge intensifies. Use your breath to immerse yourself in whole-body sensations and absorb the love offered by your lover. Use your sexual energy to nourish your own soul connection and that with your lover. If you can manage a simultaneous orgasm, the meditation at the moment of orgasm will be much more powerful.

- Let the energy pour through your body, into every cell. Together you and your partner are a vibrating ball of energy, suffused with erotic excitement.

Visualizing bliss during lovemaking

As you make love, imagine that you are generating bliss through intercourse. You can imagine bliss as sparks of light, from fireworks or a crackling fire, or you can visualize bliss as phosphorescent water glittering in the night-time ocean, released as the sea water surges past your swimming limbs.

Immerse yourself totally in the experience of joy in

order to feel this bliss. Traditionally, in Tantra, bliss is depicted as drops of golden nectar which stream down from your forehead through your body, bathing you in nourishing sustenance.

- Imagine that as you have intercourse a light, frothy golden foam arises from churning your genitals together. Let this golden foam rise up both your bodies, bathing your whole bodies in golden bubbles.
- As your united bodies are coated in this golden nectar, let it drip back down your body. Feel the drips touching your skin and take in the refreshing essence which is as soft and gentle as morning dew. Absorb it through your skin. Bathe in it. This is the essence of bliss.

Visualizing the lotus during lovemaking

You can use any image that appeals, such as two bodies of light absorbing each other or two pools of water

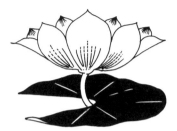

merging. Traditional Indian imagery depicts this merging as a single lotus flower blossoming above the crown of your two heads, at the moment of synchronized orgasm. You can use this visualization during sex, or at the moment of orgasm. The sitting-up position during lovemaking facilitates this as you can rest your heads together or allow your brows to touch.

- Imagine the channels of energy inside your two bodies rising and intertwining above your head in a great ball of energy.
- Whichever image you use, you can simultaneously visualize your energy-bodies interpenetrating.

Sharing vision

Vision-sharing is all about discussing your fantasies in order to formulate a vision that you can work towards attaining.

Discuss how your relationship would be, in an ideal world. Imagine it in detail – how would your sex life be? How would you like to be connected emotionally? How would you be spending your time, together and apart? Use the shared aspects of your fantasy to design a model for your ideal relationship. In designing this model, you can work towards attaining it. Sharing your vision with your partner also strengthens your spiritual connection.

Having a shared vision as a couple is having an image of how you would like your world to be. In the process of defining your shared vision, you can take the opportunity to rest in this novel perception of reality together.

Creating a vision also gives you access to a potent source of inspiration. This vision shapes your intent; it illuminates your path and helps you to make appropriate decisions so that your life flows in accordance with it.

Vision of bliss

This is an aspirational exercise to help you bring visionary qualities into your relationship. Here you use a joint meditation during which you sit and bring the image into your mind, reliving the details of the fantasy in order to develop your sense of vision. This isn't escapist nonsense, but a way of holding an ideal image in your awareness, providing a model against which to measure your own daily behaviour.

To create a vision, channel your thoughts and intentions with visualizations. Visualizing helps to actualize your image of your ideal with the joint body of your relationship – this is the energy-body that you create through doing Tantra exercises together *(see Step 1, page 48)*. When you visualize energy flowing freely throughout the different facets of your being, it helps make it happen in reality. Once you are able to call up an image, you can use your vision to create a template for your life and how you want it to be.

- Turn your attention to the area between your eyes. This is the chakra, or energy centre known as your third eye, the home of your inner vision.
- Together, create a joint vision that you can both hold in your mind's eye. For instance, call up a mental image of the two of you holding hands, walking together in a lush landscape; or a dreamed-of project, where you visualize the happiness and energy sparking between you as you share a sense of excitement and achievement. If you have children, include them in your vision too. Paint a picture of how you want your relationship to be. Imagine every detail; feel the quality of your togetherness.
- Imagine that you are living your vision.

Inner Vision

Integrating your divine sexual experience with a spiritual understanding brings a deepening of bliss. In Tantric terms, the depth of your understanding is related to the activity of your third-eye energy centre (between your brows). The third eye refers to a third source of vision – one of deeper insight based on comprehending your experience in a holistic way. Insight is also fed by developing your compassionate awareness. When you perceive the essence of your life, your lover and your own sexuality, and respond from your own essential nature, you express insight – an intuitive understanding of your relationship with the world around you. Intuition is about having a non-intellectual knowledge of the world gained through direct experience.

Intuition arises when you experience the world as mysterious – when you stop trying to pin life down, you can let the mystery arise. Your sexual relationship also benefits from fostering a sense of mystery. When you stop attempting to control your relationship you can allow it to unfold. You simply concentrate on remaining responsive. Don't take your partner or your sex life for granted. Take an open and aware stance toward your relationship. Expect the unexpected. With this attitude, you can take pleasure in the unknowability of existence.

Honouring the divine

In order to build a body of bliss *(see page 319)* a key practice is to focus on the essential nature of your partner as a god or goddess. Try to see your partner as divine, to encourage the transcendent aspects of your relationship.

Bliss is not a separate entity. A sense of separation is foreign to the Tantric world view – it is a fundamentally Western attitude to place things in oppositional relation to each other. Our cult of individualism encourages people to pursue their own goals regardless of the effect on their community. Tantra sees this as one of the causes of a sense of alienation, or separation between the self and others. When individuals only pay attention to their own needs without taking responsibility for others, they end up feeling cut off, lonely and isolated. This inevitably results in deep misunderstanding and conflict.

As humans we have a profound need for connection and understanding. By seeing the divine within yourself and your partner, you acknowledge the availability of bliss as your right. You merge with the universe. You can be at one with yourself, your beloved and the wider world through blissful love.

Imagine yourself as a deity

Sometimes, we go about our lives feeling beleaguered and lost, unaware that our real nature is divine. Your nature is the same as everything else in the world: divine. Accept that divinity is all around you as well as

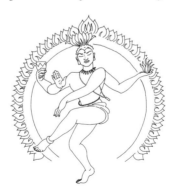

within you. Once you discover that bliss is located within yourself, you won't have to keep looking for it in someone or something else.

As Tantric Buddhists say, our true nature is already perfect. They describe our nature as a clear stillness and compassionate heart. This meditation allows you to uncover that nature as divine.

It develops a sacred view of all life and places you at the heart of creation. Your deepest essence is inseparable from the sacredness of the world around you.

By visualizing yourself as a deity, your inherent nature can flow out in unity with others. Choose a deity that inspires peace and love within you. Accepting your true nature as divine allows you to develop the qualities that you associate with that divinity.

- Sit upright with your legs loosely crossed. Lie your hands on your knees. Close your eyes and focus your attention inside, on your breath.
- After a few minutes of sitting quietly, call up the image of yourself seated cross-legged in your mind's

eye. See a small image of yourself sitting just in front of your forehead.

- You are clothed in the raiment of a divine form, and have a calm, peaceful demeanour. Your face and body radiates grace and beauty.
- Feel the love emanating from this being of pure light. The love bathes everything around you.
- Know that you are this divine being.

Be a divine lover

As a divine lover you approach your partner with a sense of your own fullness and perfection, rather than a sense of inadequacy or need. Through investing yourself with the aura of the divine, you can transform the atmosphere and quality of your lovemaking.

In order to draw on a source of sacred power during lovemaking, visualize yourself as a deity making love to your consort. Every gesture is sacred – every touch, every moment of your lovemaking.

- Start by closing your eyes and sitting in meditation for several minutes. As you breathe in, imagine that you are drawing in the divine attributes of the universe with your breath. Let holy breath enter your lungs. Let divine light fill your being. Let fiery warmth permeate your being. In your mind's eye, see yourself fill with these attributes.

- Alternatively, you can use the Tantric technique of imagining that you are whichever god you would like to be. Imagine yourself as the Lord of Creation, full of power and energy, or as a goddess, brimming with creativity and dynamism. Embrace the positive qualities of the deity and make them your own.

- Once you feel imbued with the presence of divinity, turn to your mate and imagine him or her as your consort. Approach them with power and grace. Enfold them in this sacred moment.

Divine sex: making love as a god and goddess

Tantra has its roots in the matriarchal practices of Hindu India. It encourages you to honour your sexual relationship as a mirror of the divine relationship between the primordial couple responsible for the act of creation, Shakti and Shiva.

The Tantric concept of bliss is often depicted as the goddess and god in sexual rapture, symbolizing the unification of energy and conscious awareness. In sexual rapture, two bodies and souls merge into one. From this ecstatic union, the bliss of pure joy arises.

Making love as if you are the divine couple reinstates bliss as your birthright. Become a god and goddess during your lovemaking.

- Prepare a sacred space by arranging a temple of love for your lovemaking *(see Bedroom bliss, Step 3, page 111)*.
- Spend some time in meditation, imagining yourself as a god or goddess, robed in glory and power.

- When you feel imbued with sacred qualities, imagine your lover robed as a deity, in their splendour and energy. In your mind's eye, see the light of their divine energy pouring from them.

- Visualize yourself and your partner as goddess and god. You can use an illustration from this book to create an image, or gaze at a statue or photo of a Tibetan god and goddess entwined in the act of love. Then close your eyes and imagine you are becoming that god and goddess. Visualize yourselves as the supreme deities in the generative act of creating all manifestations in the world.

- Slowly open your eyes and gaze at your partner, seeing them as you did with your eyes shut. Let their form take on a radiance and serenity that comes from their essential nature.

- Acknowledge each other as divine by the way you look at each other. You may like to give each other a flower. Approach each other as if your lovemaking is for a magical rite.

- Let your desire for your partner be within the image of a god and goddess making love. Let the spirit move you. Make love as if a god and goddess were making love through your bodies.

Radiant light meditation

Meditation connects you with yourself as the source of unconditional love, and enables you to share this with your partner. Mystics describe the true nature of reality as divine love.

Bliss is both inside you and outside you. The purpose of meditation is to ensure that your inner state is a continuum of the outer reality of bliss.

Identifying with divine energy expands your experience of yourselves. Use this light meditation to become light and ethereal, dancing freely in space like molecules of joy. Let go of the solidity of your physical bodies, and see yourselves as composed of radiant light (traditionally, bliss is described as nectar or light). If your partner is your soul mate, you can create a joint energy-body. This body is called the body of bliss.

- While you are in your partner's arms, relax into a meditative state in which your awareness of bodily boundaries evaporates. See yourselves as two bodies composed of light that naturally merges and blends together.

- Let yourself open and dissolve into your partner's energy. Experience your entwined energy-bodies as part of the endless light from the infinite number of suns in the universe. Infinity is not frightening – it is vast and timeless. There are no boundaries, and therefore nothing to restrict you or limit your bliss.

The jewel in the lotus

In Tibetan Tantra, the sacred name for intercourse is the jewel in the lotus. The penis is the jewel and the vulva is the lotus. Tantrists believe that having the penis inside the vagina balances and harmonizes your energy, and that lovemaking itself produces compassion in the form of the woman's sexual juices.

- Once you are both highly aroused, take up the yab-yom sexual posture (with the woman sitting on the man, who is sitting cross-legged on the floor, supported by cushions). As always in Tantric lovemaking, the woman chooses the appropriate moment to guide her partner's penis inside her. Delaying entry is very important – the more time you spend on other methods of connecting and stimulating each other, the more enjoyable intercourse will be by the time you get there. Once her vagina is moist and juicy, she receives his penis as an instrument of dynamic male energy. He enters her vulva as the source of creative female energy.

- Experiment with different styles of intercourse: try short strokes, deep penetration or using small thrusting movements with the penis deep inside – without pulling out. Try sweeping the cervix with your penis, rotating your pelvis and gently rocking your hips back and forth. Small movements can be surprisingly pleasurable.

- Try different angles of penetration such as angling forward, pressing your partner's pubic area and clitoris as you push inside.

- Explore using your pelvic muscles, separately and in unison. If a woman's vaginal muscles are very strong she can pleasure her partner with squeezing. Try withdrawing to the entrance of the vagina, then your partner can squeeze her pelvic muscles to draw you inside. Staying still inside and squeezing your love muscles feels very good after you've already had one orgasm.

Joy

Joy is an emotional state; it arises from your core being when you are in touch with the wonder of being alive. Joy arises spontaneously, whereas happiness is transient. Happiness is fleeting, because it is usually attached to particular conditions being just right. When things go wrong, you become unhappy. Joy is the quality of being a conscious human being. Joy is an innate quality that arises as your energy is cleansed and focused on deeper states of being.

- You can get in touch with joy by letting go of distractions. Lighten up by letting go of negative feelings or any emotional baggage you are carrying around.
- To get in touch with your capacity for joy, see yourself as an energy-being. The purpose of your relationship is to give each other joy, letting your beloved find joy in your body as well as in their own.
- When we feel this joy dawning we tend to cling on to moments of fulfilment because we are haunted by their ephemeral nature. We try to freeze such experiences, or possess them where we can. Our grasping, restless minds create a pervasive sense of dissatisfaction. Buddhists hold that imperfection, dissatisfaction and incompleteness are inevitable. In order to find peace and contentment, we need to learn to stop clinging.
- Contact your innate sense of joy by concentrating on what is happening now. The ultimate goal of bliss in lovemaking depends on a subtle unfolding of your capacity for joy. The way you make love depends on the degree to which you can access joy.

Joy in lovemaking

The first sign of joy during lovemaking is in your smile, a sign of the happiness that emotional intimacy brings.

The second stage of joy is its deepening through your gaze, when you look at your partner and see them as god-like.

The third stage of joy is in the consummation of your sexual attraction and desire through lovemaking.

The ultimate Tantric goal is 'innate joy', when you enter the bliss that follows lovemaking.

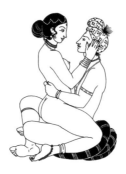

- Start your lovemaking by gazing at each other, letting your love light up your face. Let a smile play on your lips as you take delight in the presence of your lover. Look at their radiant form and see them as a being of light. As you watch, the light becomes suffused with pink, the colour of love, and then deepens into red, the colour of lust. Feel the heat of your own sexual fire kindle in your pelvis.

- Let the heat spread from your pelvis, thighs and genitals up your body. You can use your hand and your breath to sweep or draw the sensations up from your abdomen into your heart. Focus on opening your heart, allowing a sense of joy to permeate your being as you gaze at your partner. The play of emotions between you expresses itself in the variety of your play and the way you explore each other's bodies. Let your face soften and smile if you are enjoying the process.

- As you come together in intercourse, focus on drawing blissful feelings into the crown of your head where they blend together like two flames. The heat of your lovemaking will brighten this flame, which sometimes ebbs and then intensifies again.

- After lovemaking, remain in the warmth of the embers of your passion.

Body of enjoyment

You have a body of enjoyment as well as the energy-body that permeates your physical body. This body of joy is full of brilliant white light. It is nourished by joy and happiness. In feeding your body of joy, you fill it with the true nature of reality – bliss. If you identify yourself with your enjoyment-body, you can experience joy in all its intensity and power.

You can use this exercise together or as a solo meditation while lying alone.

- Imagine your body filling with a delicate, fine quality of joy arising from the centre of your being. This centre could be located in your pelvis, if you are full of sexual charge, or it could be in your solar plexus, where your abdomen rises and falls as you breathe; it could be in your heart if you are full of love for your partner. Wherever it is, let joy emanate from this area, filling your body with a subtle light energy.

- Imagine the energy taking on the quality of light, getting brighter and brighter until your body sparkles.

Merge into desire

Ecstasy is not just about a peak sexual experience. The word means moving away from stasis or stagnancy into flow. Sacred sex is about entering the flow of energy between the two of you. The more deeply you connect, the more ecstasy you can achieve.

When you are making love from a place of desire, your sense of separateness dissolves. You are no longer trying to meet each other's sexual and emotional desires. Instead you both merge into desire.

- Use gentle stroking for pleasurable sensation anywhere on the body. Through your fingertips, absorb the flesh of your beloved. Allow your skin to melt into their softening skin. Kiss, letting your breath mingle. Listen to the life flowing through their lungs and heart with their breath. It may be a quiet breath, or it may be passionate and excited. As you mingle your breath, relax your body into your partner's. Melt into each other, each lost in the other's mouth, breathing each other, becoming each other, becoming one.

- Allow yourself to dissolve so that you no longer know whose body belongs to whom, or which part of you is you. Who is man and who is woman no longer matters, just the smooth, taut skin. Let the boundaries of your body dissolve.

Variation

You can synchronize your chakras, the energy centres located up and down your spine *(see page 51)*, or circle your breath between you while holding hands *(see page 309)*.

- To circulate your breath, have your right hand facing upward, covered by your partner's cupped left hand. Imagine breath passing through your heart and streaming down your hand and into that of your partner.
- Totally merge with your experience of being with your partner. Let the walls of your separation disintegrate. Allow your body to soften, releasing any tension, holding or resistance. Soften so much that the boundaries of your separate bodies dissolve.
- Let your heart fill with energy. Let this overflow into your partner.

Erotic sensitivity

Rather than pursuing more stimulation, Tantra is concerned with experiencing more sensitivity. As you work through the Tantric practices in this book, eventually you will find that you don't need to do anything to stay connected with your partner.

When you're with your partner, relax, breathe, soften and be present to the moment. When you feel the energy charge between you building sexually, you can expand, literally letting your body take up more space. Tantrics encourage expansion by visualizing the sexual energy spreading upwards from your genitals and permeating the heart and the crown of your head.

Concentrate on letting the eroticism suffuse your whole body so that you can have a whole-body orgasm (*see page 283*). The energy of orgasm can spread from your genitals, into your whole body.

Relaxing into orgasm

Relaxing into orgasm is like falling into a flowing stream rather than directing it with your mental power. In fact, the less mind control the better, as Tantra is all about stepping out of the mind.

Staying relaxed while sexually aroused allows you to receive erotic energy from your partner.

In order to build up toward an orgasm, most people tense the muscles, especially around the thighs and pelvis.

In energetic terms, tension means that you contract inward, making it harder for energy to flow through your body. Relaxation implies expansion – allowing your erotic energy to spread throughout your whole body.

- Feel the pleasure of your emotional and sexual connection with your partner. Visualize your heart opening with love and sustain this loving mood throughout.
- Try to stimulate your partner a little and then stop, allowing them to focus on the sensations in their body without having to get on with doing the next thing. Gaze lovingly at your partner, enjoying their pleasure and the pleasure that you are granting them.
- Use blended stimulation of the pearl (clitoris) or penis, plus nipples, earlobes, toes, feet, back of the knees and inside of the elbows. While you are doing this, spread the energy through the body in long, light, smooth strokes. Concentrate on the area of the heart, pushing energy from the genitals toward the heart.
- When you are very aroused, practise sinking into a state of deep relaxation, breathing deeply yet slowly.

As you soften your body, soften emotionally and reach out in love. Concentrate on the movement of energy generated by your heart connection, as well as your erotic excitement, as you make love.

- When you feel your muscles are about to contract, try to relax them rather than striving for orgasm. If you can't reach orgasm without tensing your buttocks and thighs, try to let one or two contractions occur in your usual way, and then stop making any effort. Surrender to the pleasurable sensations in your body.

- Help yourself to relax by breathing slowly and deeply. Relax your abdominal muscles. Let yourself hover on the edge of your pleasure for as long as possible. Feel yourself on the edge for some time.

- Take turns during lovemaking. One of you pleasure the other right to the edge of your orgasm, then stop and swap roles. Keep approaching the edge of orgasm and retreating several times.

- Once you and your partner become attuned to one another, you will no longer think about who is pleasuring whom, and who is on the edge. You will both relax into a hovering state of intense pleasure in your sensations, rather than strive for a climax.

Breathing together

Regular meditation, prayer and ritual practice nurture your relationship with the divine, bringing it firmly into your relationship. It is good practice to always prepare your bedroom for lovemaking; lighting candles and incense and choosing appropriate music as well as anything else you might need later. You are setting the scene for breath meditation.

Radiant energy meditation

This meditation opens your energy through the crown of your head to connect with divine love.

- Sit in half-lotus, dove-tailed or yab-yom *(see page 167)*. Close your eyes and allow your breath to fall into a slow, steady rhythm, together. Synchronize your breath, so that you resonate with each other's body rhythm.

- Imagine that you are opening the crown centre right at the top of your head, the gateway to the transpersonal realm. Each of you imagines white light streaming in through the crown of your head. Each time you breathe in, imagine drawing this light down to the base of your pelvis. As the light fills your pelvis, hold your breath for a moment, allowing it to permeate your being. If you find it easy to visualize, try to imagine this stream of white light expanding out to fill your whole being, illuminating your body so that it becomes a radiant energy-body.

- Release your breath slowly, while your energy-body remains illuminated by your breath.

- Focus on the sexual energy in your genitals, allowing the white light to concentrate there, becoming golden in colour. Imagine that you are drawing this golden light from your genitals and pelvis with your breath, along the column through the centre of your body. As it moves up toward the crown of your head again, imagine this golden light flooding the energy centres located at your heart, your throat and your brow (third eye). Then visualize the light streaming out of your crown, to merge with the light streaming out of your partner's head.

- Visualize the energy streaming out of the crown of both your heads pooling and uniting. Create a joint body, which can look like a rainbow-body of light fanning out above both your heads.
- See yourselves as radiant beings surrounded in a rainbow of light, linked to the divine.
- Let divine love wash through you both.

The afterglow: post-coital bliss

This is an important time for going deeper into your emotional and spiritual connection. After an experience of uniting and merging as one body, you have had a taste of what it is like to let go of your separate self and merge with something greater. According to Tantra, this is the ultimate nature of existence. The dimension of bliss is always there, if only you can tap into it. After making love, abandon yourself to the loving connected-ness that is the lived experience of bliss.

Deepening the bliss

Post-coital meditation ensures that you remain deeply connected to your partner, even after the delights of lovemaking are over. Enhance sexual bliss and turn it into an experience of bliss; once bliss arises in you, you discover that maintaining it is not dependent on external conditions. As you are in a very open mode during Tantric sex, this is the perfect moment in which to maxi-mize your openness and encourage it to stay.

During Tantric sex you will also have approached an altered state. Meditating afterwards consolidates that experience, helping you to integrate it into your daily life.

• In your post-orgasmic bliss, lie together with your heart wide open, full of love for your partner. It is important to remain physically close after orgasm, to deepen the bonding process. Leave your penis inside the vagina so that your love juices are mixed and energy blends.

- Allow yourselves to fall into a state of deep relaxation, without going to sleep. Alternatively, you may be in a state of non-thinking and emptiness or a state of bliss. Lie together, imagining that you are one united energy-body. Cocoon your lover in the embrace of love.

- Relax and deepen your breathing. Imagine your unified body wrapped in a ball of golden light. Breathe in as one body, exhale as one body.

- Imagine that you are floating in the universal heart of your beloved, feeling deeply connected.

Inspiration for your relationship

Commitment

Problems of commitment are endemic in contemporary society, because of the damaging effects of a lack of intimacy in early family relationships, and the bruising experiences of careless sexual relationships before maturity.

Lack of commitment damages a relationship. If you feel ambivalent and can't manage to express your appreciation of your relationship and don't intend to stay with your partner, you should leave. Commitment is necessary to allow your relationship to grow and move forward on the spiritual path. Without commitment, you will be wracked by emotions like uncertainty and lack of trust. These negative emotions distract you from the task of increasing awareness and openness toward others. A commitment grounds your intention to pursue the spiritual path together; it means honouring your obligations rather than leaving if the going gets tough. Discuss your mutual intention to carry on dealing with emotional issues in spite of the temptation to give up.

Commitment also implies making it a priority to bring more mutual pleasure into your relationship. This means honouring any agreements that you make to practise exercises in this book together. Consider making a commitment to doing some practices from each of the seven Steps to test the possibility of making your relationship the cornerstone of your mutual development – for example, you might want to dedicate forty days to this. This will give you a chance to experience the change Tantra can bring about in your love and sex life. You will deepen your understanding of what your relationship involves, incorporating this wisdom into your being.

Heart meditation

Use this simple meditation to foster a heart connection. It helps you to nurture loving feelings and open your heart to your lover. If you find it difficult to use visualization techniques and prefer something more concrete,

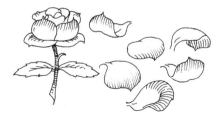

you can meditate while looking at a piece of rose quartz. Spend several minutes a day doing this meditation, sitting quietly or lying down in a relaxed position. If you are doing it with your partner, you can visualize the cocoon around both of you.

- Imagine your body wrapped in a ball of golden light, like a cocoon. Then, imagine a translucent pink light, the soft colour of rose quartz crystal, in the heart area of your chest.
- Let the rose light gradually permeate your whole body, and expand to colour the golden ball pink.

Affirmation practice

It is important to remind yourself that you are with your partner through your own free choice.

Your partner is not forcing you to remain in the relationship, regardless of the ways in which they express their attachment to you. Each day, you choose to stay.

According to your own deeper wisdom, your partner is the most appropriate person for you to be with right now. Use your own positive affirmations to make the most of the opportunities that your relationship offers you for growth. Through your relationship you can increase self-knowledge and build greater intimacy.

Because actions and emotions follow intentions, make it an intention to honour and respect your partner to create a relationship that brings out the best in both of you.

Here are some affirmations that you might like to use.

We will treat each other with mutual respect and honesty.

We are free to be together.

We honour the love between us.

We prioritize pleasure.

We glorify our sexuality.

Anniversary celebration

To celebrate another year of commitment to your partner, treat them by doing everything they want for a whole day, or a weekend if you can get away together. Indulge your lover in every way you can think of – you could begin by creating a Tantric environment in which to relax and have fun *(see Bedroom bliss, page 111)*. You may want to follow the exercise on page 127, in which you essentially do whatever your partner wants.

Remember to attune yourselves at the start of this time together *(see Step 2, page 66)*.

Love as service and devotion

The path of love involves service and devotion. Allow yourself to be a source of happiness, love and comfort for your partner. Make a gift of yourself to your partner, in the name of love.

Through giving, the sense of separation is eclipsed for both of you. Your sexual attraction gives rise to caring, loving, devotional qualities, grounding these in acts of everyday selflessness, such as when you put your partner first. Performing devotional acts shows your partner that you cherish them, allowing them to receive your love in a way they probably never have before.

Worshipping your lover as your soul mate, or beloved, means that you worship the divine in them. The divine stands for the inherently lovely, lovable and loving in human nature. Both of you are already inherently divine, and seeing each other in this light helps you to let go of petty squabbles and power-struggles in order to create a more loving union.

This is not a one-sided game. Both of you can be selfless and giving to each other.

A flower ritual for devotion

In this ritual, you make offerings of flowers or other beautiful objects to your partner while you visualize them as a deity. You will also need to think about a god or goddess with whom you feel an affiliation – a spiritual being who embodies peace and joy to you. This may be Chenrezig, the Tibetan buddha of compassion; or a Hindu deity such as Ganesh, the elephant-headed god of wisdom. You could use a divine or angelic form from your own religious tradition.

- Close your eyes for a few moments and imagine your chosen deity. Visualize them sitting in front of your forehead, clothed in fine garments, their body and gestures inspiring you with their beauty and love.
- Open your eyes and see the image of this divine being superimposed on the form of your lover. As you continue to look at your lover, imagine that the two beings are merging; your lover and the image of the god or goddess that you have called up. See how your lover's body radiates tranquility and joy. Notice how their smile is both accepting and loving. See how the light of the god or goddess fills their being.
- Visualize that you make offerings to your lover as a deity: a single lotus flower, a blossom, a jewel.

- Feel how blessed you are to be in their presence. Open up to the quality of the spiritual power invested in them by the god. Embrace the peace and energy that this image gives you.

Foot massage

A simple foot massages allows you to serve your partner with devotion. To begin, first prepare the room as your temple-space for the night: cleanse it with fresh water, scattering rose petals, or cleanse the air with burning sage. Light candles or incense before welcoming your beloved, seating him or her comfortably and offering water laced with herbs or fruit. Offer your partner flowers and perfumes, and dainties such as honeyed yoghurt or nuts and raisins.

- Prepare a warm bowl of slightly salty water for your lover to soak their feet in. Seat them comfortably in front of a single candle flame. Let them sit quietly in meditation while you go to prepare some food for later, making it with devotion.

- After fifteen or twenty minutes, give your lover a glass of water to drink (for purification) and kneel before them to dry your lover's feet with a towel. Dry their feet tenderly, and thoroughly, between their toes.
- Place a towel over your thighs and let their your partner's feet rest on your lap. Anoint their feet with massage oil or almond oil, perfumed with an essential oil of your choice *(see Step 3, page 114)*. Massage gently at first, then more firmly, exploring all the different parts: the instep, the toes, between the toes, the soles and Achilles heel. Experiment with different strokes and pressures, using your fingertips and palms.

Surrender

Surrendering means letting go of attachment and trusting the universe. In order to let the transpersonal in you need to let go of your attachment to your individual identity: you release your smaller identity to become part of something bigger. As you discover the immensity of energies you are part of, you connect with universal forces and energies – the qualities of the divine. Once you have glimpsed the possibilities of deeper connection, you may long for direct access to that experience. Your longing for oneness leads to complete surrender.

Centring prayer

If you long to feel the presence of bliss in your life, you can use this simple meditation to turn your longing into a prayer of authentic presence. You can use a key word to help you focus your attention, such as repeating the word 'love' almost like a sigh of love – the way you say the word is like a murmur of love. This meditation is a way of orienting your being toward love.

- Settle down quietly with a well-supported straight spine.
- Close your eyes, and turn your attention to the spark of divine energy that you feel within. Let this presence

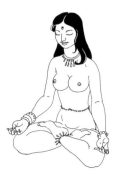

move within you. Turn yourself toward this loving presence, and allow it to fill your being.

- Simply observe the sensations that arise as a result of orienting yourself toward love. Let this energy do whatever it wants, and go wherever it wants in your body.
- Use the word 'love', speaking it inside or out loud to help return your awareness to the presence of love as a vital principle.

Allow yourself to exist without erecting any barriers to this presence of love – you need not feel overawed by it.

Surrendering to the manifestation of the divine in your life means not holding back. Meditation is the door through which you enter this radically transformed sense of reality.

The goal of meditation is to clear the intellectual and emotional garbage that you have accumulated over your lifetime. This allows space for more positive impressions to enter your awareness.

Your relationship is perfect

Think about intimate partnership as the perfect vehicle for your spiritual growth. The issues that arise in a relationship always provide an opportunity to learn something about yourself and to grow. If you approach problems in this positive way, they immediately become smaller problems. Rather than try to change your partner's behaviour, you work on refining your own awareness. Your lover reflects you; accept that what you see in your relationship mirror has some truth, rather than fall into the trap of denial, projecting your issues onto your partner.

Respect the partner that you have chosen to be with, because they are perfect for you right now: you can waste precious energy wondering if you're with the right person rather than redirect this energy into a positive learning experience. Surrender to your partner and to your experience, and ultimately to love. When you do this, you see the perfection of your love in spiritual terms.

Surrender your small notion of who you are to become part of something greater. In losing your personal identity, you gain a universal identity *(see also Surrender, page 356)*. Become one with your lover and the world around you. In becoming one you heal a sense of wounding, separation and alienation. You become whole.

Let your lover be your sexual teacher

Ask your lover to initiate you into the mysteries of lovemaking. In Tantra, the woman is seen as a sexual initiator. The woman initiates her partner by taking the lead during this lovemaking session. She determines when you start to make love, and the pace and the style of it. She determines whether you go on to have intercourse or not. During intercourse, she makes love astride her partner and actively takes her own sexual pleasure.

- Start by worshipping your lover *(see page 352)*.
- Let them initiate you into the mysteries of your sexual relationship.
- Be guided by them. Follow their suggestions when starting to make love. Let them teach you from the accumulated wisdom of their body and soul. Cultivate an attitude of keenness to learn their sexual secrets.
- Let them guide your hands and instruct you in the arts of lovemaking.
- Feel safe, and trust your lover to look after you sexually.

A goddess meditation

This is a meditation for both men and women, in which you imagine yourself as a goddess. In identifying with a female deity men are nourishing their feminine side. In Tantra women are seen as active and dynamic, while men are calm and aware. Use the goddess meditation to identify with your passionate sexual nature – regarded as feminine. In India, the goddess Shakti stands for the creative principle in life and she is depicted as a fiery dancing goddess, ringed by the flames of ever-changing life.

- Visualize yourself as a goddess, who represents your innermost being.
- Imagine that your body is entirely red, which is the colour of life, lust and passion. Meditate on this image of yourself in order to realize the essential divinity of your sexuality.
- A way to turn around your usual way of thinking is to believe that it is the deity who is meditating, rather than you – she uses you as a vehicle through which

she expresses herself. If you can enter this state of mind for the duration of the meditation, you will get even more benefit from it.

Imagine you are your partner

There is a real need to explore the sexuality of the opposite sex. Bringing an awareness of what it might be like for your partner when he or she is faced with trying to satisfy both your sexual and emotional needs is often a healing experience. Try this cross-gendered perspective on lovemaking.

- For men, take note of what your woman says about sexual experience. Listen to her suggestions in order to enhance your lovemaking. Imagine what it might feel like to be a woman and experience your caresses. What does your lovemaking feel like? What is it like to feel your penis enter? It is important for a man to be able to open up to a woman's energy during lovemaking and emotionally connect with her, rather than going after his own phallic pleasure – or being so busy doing things to try and stimulate her that she doesn't feel that he is properly connected.

- For women, imagine how it feels to be your partner and be expected to bring you to sexual fulfilment.

In Tantra, sexuality is depicted as feminine. Many women respond to the Tantric approach to lovemaking because it resonates with their own approach. In ordinary sex the man enters the woman's body, but in Tantric sex it is the woman's energy that permeates the man. Qualities of sensitivity, taking time and feeling close and loving will bring you closer to a feminine experience of bliss.

Bliss meditation

- Lie in your lover's arms, sinking into a heartfelt embrace. Allow yourself to merge with your partner in love.
- Sense the love pouring through you both and bask in

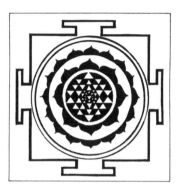

its abundance. Rest in their arms. Allow yourself the joy of feeling deeply loved. From this joy a feeling of lightness, clarity and intense sweetness arises: it is bliss.

- Fill both of your bodies with bliss. Let bliss flood into every tissue of your joined bodies – your head, your heart and your pelvis; your chest, shoulders and arms; your legs and feet. Let the quality of bliss become intense and consume you both.

- Let there be no space for anything else. Let there be no resistance or holding back. Let bliss pass through you like a wave of bubbles, cascading through your bodies from feet to head.

- Rest in bliss.

Heart drops

Use this simple but potent meditation to burn away obstacles to love and passion. You can return to it again and again on your Tantric journey.

- Visualize a red drop in your navel, below your belly button.
- Bring this inner fire up to your heart. Let all your concentration focus on this one point, the pulsating drop of blood in the centre of your heart. Let it beat at the rate of your heartbeat.
- Draw that red-hot energy into your pelvis, allowing that energy to burn away anything that is not aligned with your love of life, with joy, with vibrancy. Breathe in, drawing that heat into your abdomen. Imagine it

burning away any obstacles to your being fully in your passion, in your vitality.

- Visualize the red drop in your heart, turning into a flame. Allow the fire to burn in your heart, burning away any obstacles to love.
- With your out-breath, take the flame from the root of your spine to the crown of your head, concentrating the energy as it moves back down to your heart on the in-breath.
- Focusing your attention at the level of your heart, imagine that you are dissolving the flame in your heart. As you breathe, send all your love into this flame and let it spread throughout your body.
- If you are doing this meditation with your partner, let the flame spread from your body and into their body, engulfing you in the flame.
- Let go of any fear or resistance. Know that you are being purified. As you give up any toxicity, feel released by this burning flame.

Riding the wave of bliss

Tantric sexual experience goes beyond extended sexual pleasure. In Riding the wave of bliss, sexual pleasure spreads through your body and mind, altering your consciousness to put you in contact with ecstasy. Your sexual energy becomes a stream of bliss passing from your genitals through your joined bodies and out through the crown of your head, merging with the energy of the divine couple who endlessly recreate the world through their lovemaking.

You can access this awareness of life as bliss through sexual breathing and powerful visualization techniques. In this final exercise, you harmonize your sexual energies during an eyes-open lovemaking meditation, focusing on sustaining a constant connection with your partner to expand your experience beyond your wildest expectations. You weave techniques from many of the other exercises in this book into a joyful experience connecting body, heart and soul: sexual breathing *(see pages 92, 286);* delaying orgasm *(see page 263);* Heart wave *(see page 349)*

and Exploding orgasm *(see page 289)*.

- Start by creating a sensual relaxed ambience with music, lighting, candles and incense.
- Use massage or sensual touch to enliven and eroticize your bodies.
- Take time to connect with your partner, gazing into each other's eyes and synchronizing your breathing. You can concentrate on opening your sexual centre and your heart centre by directing your attention and your breath to those areas. Try doing this while in the upright sexual posture.
- The man needs to make himself comfortable on pillows in a cross-legged position that he will be able to sustain for at least half an hour. The woman sits nestled on his lap, with her legs wrapped around his waist.
- Close your eyes and tune into each other's breathing. As the woman slows her out-breath, the man slows his in-breath. Synchronize, pushing your breath faster for a few minutes, and then slower. Alternate faster breathing with periods of slow breathing. As you feel

warmth rising from your pelvis and genitals, squeeze them in a quick gasp, pulling up your pelvic floor muscles in rhythm with your breathing *(see page 160)*.

- Maintain the gasp and squeeze rhythm as your partner pleasures your genitals for some time. You can take turns pleasuring each other, letting your excitement ebb and flow according to the sexual dance between you.

- Your mouths are touching, and his jewel (penis) is inside the woman's lotus (vagina). This creates a circuit of energy, so that it can be circulated around your energy-bodies without dissipating. You can build higher and higher levels of energy while the areas of the body from which energy tends to leak are sealed.

- With his penis inside, hold the muscles firmly while breathing into your genitals. Build up your sexual heat together. He directs the heat from his penis into your pelvis. Feel the fire rising from the penis, through the vagina and into your entwined upright bodies. Slowly, the man circles his pelvis, encouraging the slow fire to snake up your spine and through the energy centres in both your bodies. Your energy is linked through your connected genitals.

- Squeeze your pelvic muscles, holding them as you both hold your breath. One of you will be holding your breath in, the other will be holding without any air in their lungs. When it's no longer comfortable, take a breath, and let your partner exhale at the same time. Hold your breath again and relax the rest of your body. Allow the energy to stream upwards through your body.

- Once you feel the energy streaming through your body you can stop holding the breath at the end of each exhalation and inhalation. Breathe naturally, with one partner inhaling as the other exhales, mouths sealing this exchange of energy with sealed lips.

- Now just let go, as you both circulate your breath through your lips and connected genitals. As your partner exhales, breathe in their warm breath, and imagine it travelling all the way down to your sexual centre. As you breathe out, send the sexual energy out through your tilted pelvis into your partner's genitals.

From there your partner will draw the energy up to the brow, between their eyes.

- When you're both feeling very aroused and on the verge of orgasm, close your eyes and roll them upwards, focusing inwards. This will delay the onset of the orgasm, building its intensity.
- When you are both ready to come, abandon yourself to a lengthy orgasm, focusing on the energy coming out of the crown of both your heads, pooling together as described on page 312. Remain joined together, gazing at each other while you relish this transcendental experience. This is bliss. Accept it and honour it.

Your sexual energy is as intense as fire: it leaps, sparks and guts. It continually changes while both giving out and absorbing energy. The Tantric view is that this active, consuming quality is the nature of reality itself. When you acknowledge your ultimate nature as fiery, you connect with your deepest self. In doing so, you begin to actively engage in the blissful love affair that is yours to enjoy with all of existence.

Index